THE FIGHT

THE FIGHT

WANTING TO GIVE UP, CHOOSING TO BE STRONG, AND THE INSPIRATIONAL PURPOSE FOR STAYING ALIVE

ANTHONY DANIELS

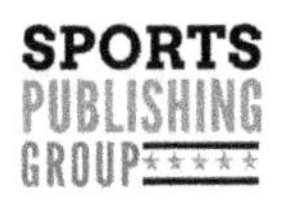

The Fight: Wanting to Give Up, Choosing to Be Strong,
and the Inspirational Purpose for Staying Alive

Published by Sports Publishing Group, Franklin, Tennessee

Edited by Ann Tatlock

Cover Design and Interior Design by Suzanne Lawing

Printed in the United States of America

978-1-734085-02-0 (paperback)
978-1-734085-03-7 (hardcover)

IN MEMORY OF

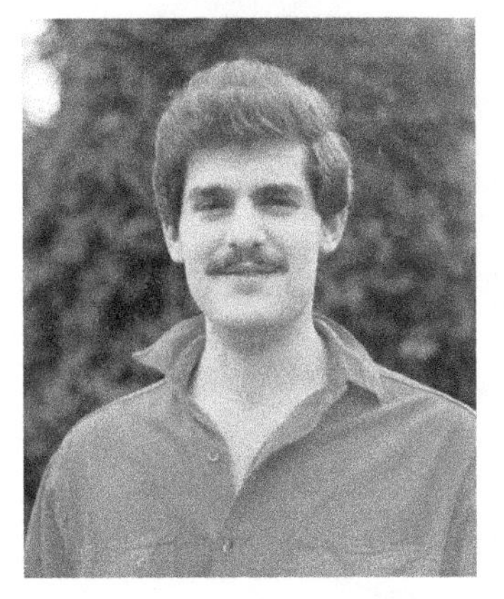

Steven Manzino

1962-2018

"He was our shining light"

DEDICATION

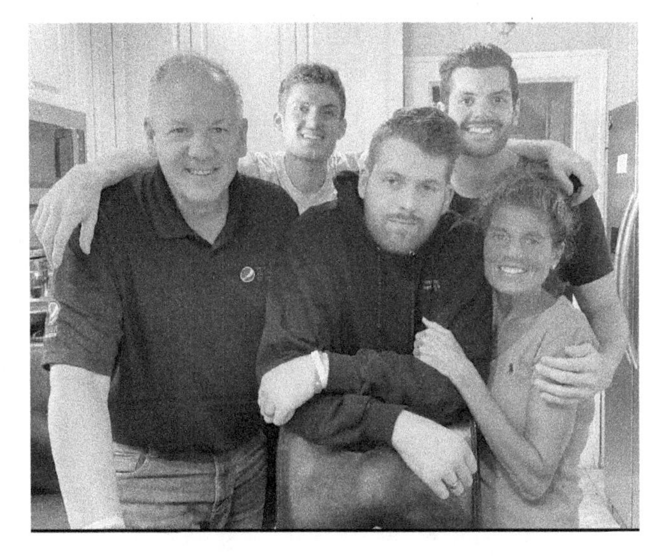

This is MY world. My heart. My love. My strength.
It all comes from you. Thank you all for never giving up on me
even when I wanted to give up on myself. This is my secret weapon.
This is my family. This is the Daniels family.

CONTENTS

Foreword

MEET ANTHONY DANIELS

Near the steps of the Philadelphia Museum of Art is a statue of Sylvester Stallone—gloved hands raised in victory—in his iconic role as boxer Rocky Balboa. The *Rocky* movies were and still are wildly popular, as everyone loves the story of the underdog who, through sheer headstrong determination, pursues his goal against all odds and wins. Watching Rocky beat Apollo Creed for the championship title leaves us feeling triumphant. Still, at the end of the film, the credits roll and we are reminded that it is all make-believe.

In your hands you're holding the incredible true story of a young man—also a boxer—who has faced insurmountable odds with that same dogged determination and who, over and over again, has met his goal and triumphed. This young man hasn't been fighting for a championship title; he has been fighting for his life.

Meet Anthony Daniels. He is a five-times survivor of Hodgkin's lymphoma, and he is currently in round 6 with this seemingly relentless opponent. For a dozen years, he has battled lymphoma, which began as a mass in his chest and has at varying times spread to his brain, hip, lungs, and spine. His doctors have predicted his death several times over. Yet, he is still alive and he is still fighting.

For Anthony, it all started with itchy feet. He was 19 years old and in his sophomore year at Fordham University in New York City at the time. For weeks he tried to ignore the irritating symptom, but the itch spread like fire to his entire body. He experienced vertigo and night sweats and had difficulty focusing his eyes. He visited a dozen doctors before he was finally diagnosed. Three days before Christmas 2010, he got the call. It was cancer.

Broadsided by the diagnosis, he underwent treatment and eventually beat the disease, only to have it return. It was then Anthony knew he had a choice. As he explains it, "I made a choice. A choice that has changed my life. I chose to be strong." He has always been an athlete, and had in fact wanted to be a professional hockey player before he was hit by a car and permanently sidelined by a broken leg. But sports continued to be his first love, and as he faced his second round of cancer treatment—both chemotherapy and radiation—he decided to take up boxing. He found a gym near his home of Ridgewood, New Jersey, and talked a hesitant trainer there into taking him on. After that, for years, he would have his treatments in the morning and be in the boxing ring in the afternoon, no matter how awful he felt.

He went on to beat cancer four more times, though every time it eventually returned. When the cancer reached his brain, he was told that he would not survive. But he did. He had to give up boxing because he could no longer take the risk of being hit in the head, but that didn't deter him. He exercised his way out of his wheelchair and began strongman training. Not surprisingly, Anthony likes to quote those famous words of Babe Ruth: "It's hard to beat a person who never gives up."

All told, Anthony has so far had about 1,000 hours of chemotherapy and over 100 units of radiation. He has had two stem cell transplants as well, but neither helped. To survive, he still needs a bone marrow transplant from a perfect-match donor. In 2015, Anthony partnered with the global organization DKMS (Delete Blood Cancer) to help find that perfect match that would keep him alive. He spoke at the 9th Annual DKMS Gala in New York City in April 2016, and did several media campaigns with Cindy Crawford and artists Pink and

Rihanna. He also appeared with actor and cancer advocate Bradley Cooper on *Good Morning America* to raise awareness of the need for bone marrow donors. Even though Anthony has so far not found his perfect match, his work has brought in tens of thousands of donors. Many of those resulted in matches for other cancer patients, which means countless lives have been saved.

In 2018, he launched the Anthony Daniels Foundation, and though much of the work had to be put on hold during the Covid pandemic, Anthony is still making plans to use his Foundation to spread his story, to raise funds for cancer patients, and to mentor one-on-one those who are presently in their own battle with the disease.

One of Anthony's dreams has been to get his story into book form so that his personal fight with cancer can be an encouragement to others. Over the course of three years, during chemo and radiation treatments, while enduring relentless pain, Anthony has pushed through it all to put words on paper. He desires to tell his readers ... to tell you ... that no matter what challenges you are facing, you can choose to keep fighting, you can choose never to give up hope, and you can choose to hold on to faith in God, knowing He has a purpose for your life even in the midst of suffering.

As our editorial team was preparing his manuscript for publication, one of the editors mentioned to Anthony that a close family member had just been diagnosed with leukemia. Anthony immediately responded, "Listen, give him my phone number and if he needs to talk, tell him to call me. I'm here for him."

That's Anthony Daniels. And here, in his own words, is Anthony's story.

~ Editorial Team, Sports Group Publishing
July 2022

INTRODUCTION

"The courage it takes to share your story might be the very thing someone else needs to open their heart to hope."

—Unknown

What's your purpose?

I know in my heart that this book is mine. We've all been through something, and our family is no different. We've been on this cancer journey for years now and my family and I have witnessed so much tragedy, including the death of my uncle. I have two younger brothers who have witnessed my cancer journey and it's been hard on them, even though they didn't have cancer themselves.

One of the things that scared me the most during this journey is the realization of how easy it would be just to quit. There's insecurity, pain, and a lot of fear. But no one had to deal with it but me. The worst part of the cancer process is that you feel like you have a gun to the back of your head every day and you're not even sure if you're going to wake up every day. This is why I feel it's so important to tell my story. I want to help others overcome their emotional and physical pain by understanding that they are not alone.

At the end of the day, it doesn't matter if I'm here to tell the rest of my story or not. We all have to face our mortality at some point and most people will never write about it. I want to tell my story to help people know that they can get through it. Mindset is everything. All that matters is that my book can help others.

God has placed a lot of angels in my path throughout this journey and many of them have helped me with this book. As you read through this, please know that it's my intention for you to take what you can from my story and use it in your own life. When I first was diagnosed with cancer, I had no idea of course that my uncle would experience the same thing. Cancer was a bond that connected us, but it was so much deeper than that.

We were the only ones who knew exactly what kind of mental and physical battle the other one was going through, and we spent every minute of every day together. He saw me at my worst and we shared painful and hilarious moments together.

When we called 911 to help my uncle in his last moments, I remember how I was too weak to lift him up off the bed. I learned so much through that experience and he taught me to manage my cancer with strength. Losing him was the worst moment of my life. Even worse than my own cancer treatments.

I have experienced more adversity than most people and my uncle is a driving force for this book. What would he say if he read it? I think of him and feel him every day. The first major surprise that I had in life was when I was a hockey player, and very athletic and strong.

I was a young athlete—and then I got hit by a car. Hockey was my life. The accident caused me to sink into a depression but I realized that I couldn't stay in a dark place. Everyone has a story, but it's your choice to change your mindset. Once I get angry, I believe that's when results happen because you're also productive, whereas feeling sorry for yourself is poison. Loneliness can set in quickly.

When you have a life-threatening disease, you realize how much you lean on those around you, even more than you ever thought you would. I'm close to my mom and she's my best friend but not everyone has that. My family helped me get through it all.

After my initial car accident, there was disappointment after disappointment because your normal life responsibilities don't just disappear when you have adversity. The adversity comes on top of whatever stress is already there.

I had relationships and goals that were ripped away from me at the last minute unexpectedly, which makes me know that I have a mission here on earth. Regardless of where you stand, you have a mission here on earth. At one point I prayed to God, "If you keep me alive, I'll tell the world about you." I knew at that time, after all my goals were stripped away, that I needed to rely on God more than ever. Whatever you're going through can be overcome, but you just have to push through it.

This book has been a healing process for me, to talk about all the scars I endured along the way and all of the healing too. My family and I have endured so much.

With all that adversity came surprising things such as confidence and wisdom. Cancer gave me pain, but it also gave me purpose.

Chapter 1

WHAT'S YOUR PURPOSE?

"The two most important days in your life are the day you are born and the day you find out why."
-Mark Twain

I was 19 years old and a sophomore at Fordham University in New York City when I was diagnosed with blood cancer. I hope your teen years were more carefree and you didn't have to experience a cancer diagnosis. I had experienced adversity before, when I was hit by a car that ended my hockey career. I'd always been an athlete and hockey was my life. Coming up against adversity for the first time, I was smacked in the face with a realization that no one could face the trial for me; I had to face it for myself.

With each adversity, no matter what it is, you're forced to fight or flight. The one thing you may not know now is that it's too easy to give up. Giving up is easy because you can face so much adversity that you lose your will to fight. I'm here to tell you not to choose to give up. The world needs you. It's not something I would've said at the beginning of my journey fighting cancer, but it's what I know now. My life purpose is to help others not give up and throw in the towel. If I can help you change your perspective from dark to light, I've won. Fighting cancer isn't nearly as hard as fighting negative thoughts. I think most of us will agree that fighting against yourself can feel frustrating and put you in a dark space, but when you fight for others, things change. My entire family has become closer than ever, but we've also all felt the hurt of loss that cancer brings. My brother, Vincent, has been heroic, and even stepped up into the caregiver role when I needed it. My mom is everything to me and has gone to the doctor appointments to ask questions, help schedule treatments, and follow up on everything involved, such as medications.

Cancer brings a lot of fear and anxiety about when the end of your life is going to be. No one wants to die young. I've always had a big drive for competition and a desire to love life full on, and I want to live my life. I force myself to believe in myself, and even though I lost 50% lung function after my first treatment, I started boxing and training. There were times I was so sick I got the crap beat out of me and there were times I won. But I trained all the time and did not allow cancer to define me. I had to find things that were mine, and I needed to fight to live. One way I have added years to my life is by helping others. Before I was sick, I was a hockey player. My biggest problem as a fifteen-year-old was that I was mentally weak when I was playing sports and I prayed to God to help me. I recall saying that I'd do anything if he would make me mentally strong. I asked for it, and I got it but I lost a lot to get it.

After I got sick, I became a patient. Life changed, and I was always forced to adapt. One year during treatment in Texas, it was so hard that every day was the worst day of my life. In 2018 I was battling blood and brain cancer and I had 47 tumors in my body. I was 147 pounds and I went to the gym and I couldn't even lift weights. I recall seeing my coach who taught me exercises in my wheelchair! I came so close to death but when I focused on staying alive that competitive drive kicked in.

Life is short. Don't spend time on the things you don't want; instead, create a life that fulfills you. I had times of pain but I never felt like giving up because I had my family to hold on to. I coach cancer patients to stay connected to this world, to find a dog, a human, or family. We all need a support system. You have to believe in yourself and if you don't, you've got to fake it until you do.

There are always curveballs in life but with danger it feels like you have them every week. I was an emotional child when I first got sick with cancer. But I knew that I had to be strong, and I drew on the strength from my parents who sacrificed their whole life for me. I decided to wake up every day and fight. It would've been easier to quit but not when you see others fighting for you. When I get sad, I try not to dwell in those emotions, and I get back up and get over it quickly. Since I was an athlete, I was very competitive and that means you never want to lose! Athletes don't go into the game or get in the ring to lose. Helping others is like a drug for me and when I can help reduce their suffering, it helps me too. I don't get in the ring to lose. I like to prove everyone wrong, and I've done that so many times during the past decade.

The hardest thing wasn't hearing that the cancer came back, but in losing the fight of the moment. My girlfriend was a professional soccer player and when I couldn't play hockey anymore, it made me feel self-conscious about myself. I started training during cancer treatments and it gave me the strength mentally to carry on. What kind of unexpected fights have you been thrown into?

We had so many unexpected events along the way and even while writing this book, we had planned on various events surrounding the launch, but a pandemic hit. This was yet another event we couldn't have prepared for. Trying to cope with the idea of dying at such a young age is hard enough, and the pandemic isolated everyone even worse. Each time I feel bad about myself I do something to strengthen my mindset and visualize success.

Chapter 2

SOMETIMES TO FOCUS WE NEED A DISTRACTION

"Being strong is a choice."

Anything you can focus on to keep you hopeful is a healthy distraction during cancer. But I didn't just envision this book helping only those of you who have a physical illness. It doesn't matter if it's a drug addiction, divorce, or depression that I can inspire others through. Pain is pain and if you read my story and take away one thing, it's: Never give up.

Cancer has brought me new friends too and several who are close friends. Helen Demestihas is one of them. I met Helen in 2013 when I was battling cancer for the second time and my only chance of survival then was to find a bone marrow donor. My brothers were a match for each other, but not for me. Helen was working at DKMS, a global organization and largest bone marrow donor center in the world. My father reached out to DKMS for assistance. It was at this time my path crossed with Helen's. Due to her extreme knowledge working with patients and her network in the community, she quickly took on the task to help me search for a donor. This was a turning point in both of our personal lives. I have always lacked trust in people and did not always make friends quickly. But with Helen, it was different. My family and I had an immediate connection.

Prior to meeting Helen in October 2013, my father shared that I had recently been in a discouraged emotional state. I was at the lowest point anyone in my family had seen me since my diagnosis three years earlier.

For the next five months of learning about me, Helen was my biggest advocate, although most of her work was behind the scenes. In the meantime, I began training as a boxer as a way to motivate myself, focusing on getting strong both mentally and physically. Despite having over 800 hours of chemotherapy and several late-night trips to the hospital, I found myself in the boxing ring directly following treatment. This was the pivotal moment when Helen approached me directly outside of my family. She asked that I team up with her to help spread my story, which she convinced me had a lot of potential to inspire and motivate other cancer patients and raise awareness to potential donors.

Together we collaborated with the National Hockey League's annual campaign "Hockey Fights Cancer," #AnthonysFight, and #GotCheeks. The success of these campaigns inspired her to go further than we had ever imagined.

When Helen left DKMS in 2015, she did not stop advocating for me. She continued to work behind the scenes to educate people on the importance of joining the registry as well as inspiring other cancer patients to believe in hope and faith. She checked in on me periodically, always willing to help any way she could. In November 2019, she reached out, inspiring and motivating me to continue where we had left off back in 2015. Our relationship is like no other. There is a lot of trust and loyalty, and more importantly we motivate and inspire each other.

I met Katharina Harf, co-founder and vice chairman of DKMS in 2015 after Helen introduced my story to her. Katharina was immediately inspired by what she heard and asked that I speak at the DKMS Annual Gala in New York City. This was the first time I had spoken to a large crowd of celebrities and prominent guests. From that moment Katharina organized global advocacy efforts to support my call to action for a bone marrow donor. I owe a lot to her for the support, passion, and immense kindness she has given to me. Katharina spent countless hours introducing my story to others, from celebrities to business and fashion leaders from all over the world. Helen and Katharina were having a brunch meeting following the gala where I was one of the guest speakers when they both approached actor Bradley Cooper, who is best known for his roles in *The Hangover Trilogy* and *A Star is Born*. They asked him to consider joining in the global efforts of DKMS.

Bradley Cooper was intrigued. He encouraged them both to keep in contact so that he could assist in #AnthonysFight. A month later, I appeared alongside Bradley Cooper on *Good Morning America,* during which he asked the viewing audience to join the registry in hopes that someone could save my life or someone like me. Within hours of the *Good Morning America* broadcast, over 5,000 people joined the registry. Unfortunately, none were a match for me. However, eight life-saving matches were found for patients that had been suffering, like me.

I was sick in bed once after chemotherapy when I got a knock on my door. It was a package from Bradley Cooper. He sent me Mike Tyson's boxing gloves that were signed and given to him by Tyson in 2010. You can imagine my excitement! He knew I was an avid boxer and even though Bradley loved the gloves he gave them away. Along with the gloves, he wrote a nice note that said he couldn't imagine giving them to anyone else. Unfortunately, the actor's life has been greatly impacted by cancer too. Cooper's father died from lung cancer in 2011.

When you lose someone to cancer it's usually after a long process of treatments, so you've prayed for them to get better and are hopeful. When they're not getting better or getting the treatment they need, it's devastating. Having the opportunity to match people with donors—there's no greater achievement in my life than giving people a second chance at their life.

I needed a bone marrow transplant and that's how I first met Bradley Cooper. My connection with Bradley, like mine with Helen's, was immediate and special. He took me to the US Open and we went to an Adele concert and hung out backstage. We would meet for lunch or dinner in New York City, and I flew out to Los Angeles to meet his family. One of the most incredible opportunities was having a small part in his film, *A Star is Born.*

Chapter 3

WHAT CANCER SHOWED ME

"God gives each and every one of us gifts. The gift I was given was the ability to fight. Whether it's for myself or someone else. I do not know how to quit. At the end of the day I will never ever give up."

One of the things cancer taught me is to fight. I think you have a choice each and every day to fight or give up and when you get a diagnosis as terrible as cancer you realize how precious life really is.

When I was young, I was scared to get a flu shot, and now I can get a shot in my neck or even surgery without flinching. I had to train my mind to feel this way. In our lives we tend to focus on our losses when we need to focus on our wins. That means developing a fight attitude and knowing that when you go into a fight, you're going to get bloody. It should be a normal part of life and you can learn from everything. Cancer taught me that anything and everything is important.

Fear is an emotion you may face, but you have to be courageous. You'll face so many emotions but you've just got to make the decision to stay strong. Another lesson cancer taught me is to keep it simple. People tend to complicate things too much. When you go through something, why wouldn't you try to get the most out of it? If you know there will be stress and pain, prepare yourself to face it and trust yourself. When my cancer came back, I felt defeated and felt like I didn't win.

If your life is perfect and you have no adversity you can't really learn too much. You need adversity to grow even more than you think is possible, and I know that if I hadn't gotten cancer, I wouldn't be who I am today. I've had an interesting, dramatic, difficult, and eclectic life and I can't be bitter about it. I can only get upset when I see what it does to my parents. Other than that, I view cancer as a gift because it's given me my purpose to help people.

Cancer has also taught me many things:

The importance of family - During traumatic times, stress has the potential to drive people apart or gather them closer. My family has saved me. The sacrifices my parents and brothers have made to keep me alive have been my biggest motivation to fight. My mother gave up her life, like any mother would do, to care for me 100% of the time for the past 12 years while I've had cancer. I call her my cancer manager. To witness the lengths she has gone to in making sure I was given the best care has been nothing less than extraordinary.

Fear - As humans, we don't like uncertainty or fear. We would rather know what we are going to experience, especially if it's life altering, than not know what's possibly pending. Because of cancer, I have lived with fear for the majority of my adult life. Will this treatment kill the cancer or will the cancer grow? Will my scan show my cancer is improving or getting worse? When I fall asleep, will I wake up? For several years, I trained myself to face my fear so I would not miss out on living.

Adversity - Adversity affects each person differently; it takes on many forms. How you choose to react when it strikes is important. In order for me to overcome hard times, challenges, and adversity I needed to face it head-on. When we are faced with something bad, we want to walk away and never deal with the situation directly. I have found with my cancer journey, building internal emotional strength and courage helps me learn from the loss with a clear mind and correctly. How do I know? As I've battled Hodgkin's lymphoma six times, along with brain, hip, and spine cancer, I've been faced with some of the biggest challenges that have tested my strength, courage, and emotional state. By making the choice to fight adversity, I was able to put on my boxing gloves after a full chemo treatment and box for hours. More than once I've boxed while in the most pain I've ever experienced from the chemo and with a temperature as high as 102. Cancer has taught me what it means to be strong. And you will never know how strong you are until it's your only option. Cancer was not my enemy; I was cancer's enemy.

You may not see it now, but adversity is actually a blessing, not a threat. It is an opportunity to prove to yourself how strong you really are. It is an opportunity to make changes you have not made if you were not forced to do so. Learning how resilient you are through adversity, trauma, or stress is something to be proud of, not ashamed.

Faith - Since my cancer diagnosis, I have learned a lot about life in general. The important things. The not so important things. Things that used to take up such large amounts of my life now seem so insignificant in the grand scheme of things. It's funny to think about how much time we spend worrying about things that don't matter. Not everyone leans on faith, especially during a time like hearing you have cancer for the first time. Faith is very personal to all of us. It's a journey and something you have to work out on your own. I was born and raised Catholic. I have spent many hours speaking to our family priest over my decade-long diagnosis. There was so much I thought I knew and so much I learned during my cancer journey. I no longer have doubts and know God has a chosen path for me.

Relationships - Numerous people with cancer have said that cancer results in true friendships. Some people feel uncomfortable talking about cancer or back away from the patient out of awkwardness or fear; it is the friends and your relationships that step up in this time of need that show true loyalty.

Chapter 4

NEVER GIVE UP

"There comes a time during that make-or-break moment.
It's in that moment when we feel like we can't fight
anymore that we have to fight even harder."

When most people face adversity, their first reaction is to give up. They decide to give in to the pain and to the mental toll it takes on your body and mind. They give up by allowing their minds to entertain all of the negative possibilities. Anyone who has experienced a cancer diagnosis will tell you that their first thought isn't "Oh, this is a great thing!" The first thought is generally about dying. About the what ifs. But if you allow yourself to get into that headspace, things quickly turn bad.

I've always loved to fight in a literal sense—in the boxing ring. The fighting makes me feel stronger and even after my cancer diagnosis I loved to get in the ring and fight. But the fight to overcome whatever obstacle you're facing is far more than a literal physical fight. The fight starts in the mind.

I love boxing and I love physical activity and it's been particularly challenging for an athlete like me to be sidelined with cancer. "The

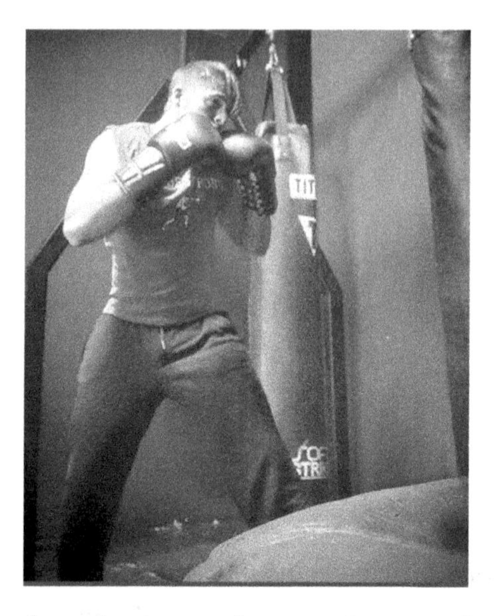

Fight" doesn't refer to boxing ... there are times you have to fight with no strength at all. There are times you have to fight for another day, fight to have faith and let God take over for you. It's not always possible to be strong in the fight.

I talk a lot in the media but also in this book about being strong. You have a choice: you can give up and lose. Or you can try to gain strength and courage in order to fight. It's important to know that even if you don't feel strong physically or mentally that you can still make the decision to fight.

While living in the Covid world has become everyone's new normal temporarily, I don't think it's going away anytime soon. I've learned to manage what is considered safe for me and what isn't. Of course, like everyone, I find living in the midst of a pandemic stressful but that is mainly due to the unknown. I would have never thought it would go past two months, and here we are, at the time of this writing, more than two years into it. A lot of good has come out of Covid. I was able to spend time with my younger brother, Michael, who in a non-Covid world lives two hours away. With the quarantine, he moved back home with us and worked remotely. He returned to his own home in

September 2020, but having him at home is still one of my favorite quarantine memories.

My mother has returned to work, which she hadn't been able to do for a year due to my health. Having her back teaching kindergarten has given me a sense of normalcy, both with Covid and my cancer. My father is still working remotely from home, but it's as if he's not even here from 8:00 a.m. to 6:00 p.m. I had over a month where I had the house to myself which allowed me to focus on my work. However, in October 2020 my grandparents (my mother's parents) sold their home in New York and moved in with us. This transition has been surprisingly simple. I was anxious about having my grandparents here 24/7 because it would just be more stress on my mother. But again, it has been going great. I've taken on cooking with my grandmother, which has now become a daily routine. I'm thinking of this as training for when I move on my own so I can cook healthy and not eat out every night.

If I had to generalize how I feel about my life right now I would say I feel appreciative. Once when I was admitted into the hospital in 2020, I honestly did not think I would be going back home. I was so sick, my fear immediately was death. Prior to getting admitted to the hospital I had so much anxiety and fear. I wasn't sleeping. I wasn't taking enough self-care. I allowed everything around me to stress me out. And I don't know exactly what was stressing me out. It wasn't anything specific. I believe it was more that my cancer was never going to leave me. If I had a pain in my leg, for example, it would keep me up all night because I couldn't help but to think it was cancer. If I had a headache, I couldn't stop thinking, "Oh God, no, my brain cancer is back." If my parents had a bad day, it would stress me out because I want them to be happy. I'd feel responsible for their bad days, whether it was another medical bill that they had to figure how they would pay (that would give me guilt and stress). If my manager, Helen, didn't have good news for me every day about my book or a plan, I would think it wasn't actually going to happen.

I struggled with thoughts that my dream of sharing my story in a book would never become a reality. That would keep me up at night. Even after Helen would constantly tell me on a daily basis that everything was going great and plans were being developed. I heard her but I didn't want to believe her. It's a defense mechanism to think things are not going to happen so that way I won't be disappointed. But it consumed me.

When I would work out, if I could only lift weights in half the pounds than the last time, I thought I wasn't getting stronger and if I'm not getting stronger the cancer is back. The anxiety kept only getting worse. So, when I was admitted into the hospital because I wasn't able to breathe, my life changed at that moment. I prayed to God if I could survive this and go home, I promised I would live life more in the moment and get help in how to control my anxiety better. I was tested for Covid. It came back negative.

They admitted me for further tests. For several days I thought this was it. I was going to die. Ironically, I was at the hospital where I was born and all I kept thinking was, "My life is going to end right where it began." Because I was having difficulty breathing, I thought maybe my lungs were infiltrated with cancer. Fortunately for me, that wasn't the case. And if that was the case, then yes, I wouldn't be here talking about this experience today.

As my oxygen and lung functions improved and tests were coming back as "no sign of cancer" or any other determinations, I was discharged and sent home. I spent a lot of time rehabbing, resting, sleeping, and making sure I focused on getting my lungs strong again. I had the house to myself most days. I'd stretch, walk, do my breathing exercises and light workouts, then rest.

I've had to work at getting better at the things I'm not as good at mentally. Like my anxiety. I've met with a therapist to help with how to cope when I feel anxious or panicked. I look at it this way: I can't do the things I want to do with the book and the Foundation—and more importantly, I can't help people who are counting on me to share my story—if I'm not healthy. So, I have to make sure I don't let what happened to me in 2020 put me in the hospital. And worse case, if it does happen again, it won't damage me emotionally like it did. I felt like I fought 12 rounds with Mike Tyson.

I really still can't believe what happened to me. It came out of nowhere and was very dramatic for me. Life really threw me a curve ball, that's for sure, and unfortunately it can't be fixed in a day—but I will get there. I'm already doing better than anyone anticipated, including myself. No more living in fear. I just have to find a way to train myself not to allow fear to take over to where I don't sleep for months consistently. I need to continue to do a lot of reading and listening to podcasts. I must have written 50+ pages in my journal so far just to figure this all out. I'm relentless when it comes to recovery, I really am. I am turning this health crisis into a gift. My message … live in the moment. Don't let what may or could or what is happening keep you from living in the moment. There is always a means to adapt or change to make your life more enjoyable to live in.

Chapter 5

THE POWER OF HOPE

"Hope is being able to see that there is light despite all of the darkness."
– Desmond Tutu

Hope has always been a part of my daily ritual. Whether it's hoping to feel better that day and not have pain. Hoping that my family and I are on the path of what we all want. Being told I was going to die quite a few times over the years really has had such a crazy effect on me. Fighting for my life and hoping I get farther and farther away from being sick is what I hope for. Training as hard as I do makes me feel a lot better physically and mentally and the better I do, the more hope I will have to live a long happy life. Hoping that every day I get bigger, stronger, faster, and most importantly, feeling very healthy. Hope for the better in every aspect. Hoping my family won't get sick or have a bad day. Hoping that I won't be sick and I will accomplish what I want for the day and get to the point where I feel closer to accomplishing my dreams. I hope for health so I don't suffer like I have. Hope gives me confidence so I know where to go in my life and be who I want to become.

I find joy the most when I'm helping people. Whether it's just jumping on a call and helping someone through a tough time or anything they need. Getting where I want physically brings me joy because of how hard it is to be big, strong, and fast when you've been sick for so many years. There are so many things that bring me joy and where it's most focused is my career. I find joy in having a job that requires me to help save lives and become the person that inspires people. Not just cancer patients but everyone. I want the world to know me and my story because I truly believe it can help people get through the toughest times in their lives. Doing my work with my team and making a plan to get there is very exciting. So it's my job to keep beating cancer over and over and to be the best me I can possibly become.

I think about all the pain I've gone through, both physical and mental. I've suffered in ways I didn't even think were possible. On one hand, that makes me so proud because I got through the suffering, but it also scares me because I know it's very possible such pain can happen at any moment. I've suffered the most mentally, dealing with thoughts of "Am I going to die today? Is today my last day or what's going to happen tomorrow?" It's a never-ending cycle and it's my job to take life one day at a time. No matter what is thrown at me, I always throw back and never give up. But when I hear the word cancer, I think of all the things that have happened to me and that makes me sad because my family had to watch it. But at the end of the day, I'm proud of my scars because it meant that cancer didn't beat me and suffering has made me strong. In every way physically and mentally I've become strong and the more I suffer the more I overcome and the stronger I become.

My hope and expectations are to help change thousands if not millions of people for the better. I've really been on one hell of a journey and it's something that's so crazy I still can't believe I came through it the way I have. My story is the one thing I'm most proud about in this world and always will be. I intend to live a long life and to accomplish everything I've wanted for many years. Being a speaker and talking around the world. Making my Foundation into something that changes lives globally. And the newest one is becoming an author and having a book (my story shared) done. A book to me is important because it's something that will last forever. There's a quote by Bruce Lee that says, "The key to immortality is first living a life worth remembering," and that's something I intend on doing whether I have cancer or not. My expectations in friends are to have a small group of friends that will be loyal and be there for me like I would for them for the rest of my life!

My expectations for my family are for them to heal and have an easier life and for them to be proud of everything I've done. Without them I wouldn't be here, it's as simple as that and I will give everything I get for the rest of my life. Now with God I intend to always stay faithful and have him part of my life as always. Years ago, when I thought I was going to die, I told God that if he kept me alive, I would be faithful to him and spread the word of my faith around the world. I want to let people know that I believe in him and that he is there and has been there for me during my darkest times.

When you have cancer, everything slows down. You're not as productive as you are normally. What steals my focus and energy and prevents me from living in the moment is when I'm in a ridiculous amount of pain.

I'm a tough guy, but the pain I feel sometimes is so severe I can't think straight. One thing that steals my energy is panic attacks. They are something I've had to deal with since my first one during my first stem cell transplant. Basically, physical things that happen only really take me away from living in the moment. I've worked very hard since I got sick to always appreciate the moment and never sway from it. But it's not easy now. The team at OnFire Books has been understanding and kind during this process as Patti or Tammy asked me questions that focus on legacy. They continue to tell me that my legacy will be documented and live on forever, and I know that's true.

A legacy is about a life well lived and a purpose completed. It doesn't have to be work. It's about your inner mission and the purpose

God has given you. Your legacy could be to change lives through your suffering, your struggles, or your experiences. What is your legacy? How do you want to impact the world? Your legacy lives on for a thousand generations.

This book is certainly a way to communicate my legacy, which is to teach people to just fight. Wake up and fight one more day. Be like a boxer and get in the ring even if you've got a bloody nose. Be mentally strong even when you don't feel physically strong.

My human experience that most defines me is how many times I've beaten cancer. It shows how I never, never give up and how I've proven no matter what I can get through anything and accomplish anything. Beating cancer is such a hard thing to do but to have beaten it five times over almost 12 years is my human experience that has defined me.

My legacy is how much I've suffered and through the times I was suffering I chose to help people first no matter what. To change lives while I was fighting for my own life is what I would say my legacy was. I was an athlete even when I was most sick. It proves you can do anything and there are no excuses. God has given me strength to do all I've done and has made me feel that he has my back. I can go through anything and accomplish anything. The way I want to change the world is for them to know that anything is possible and that all you have to do first is believe in yourself and watch how amazing you become.

Chapter 6

LEGACY

"The key to immortality is first living a life worth remembering."
- Bruce Lee

Nothing has been harder during my cancer journey than watching my uncle Steve die. He lived in our home during his illness and he and I were sick at the same time. My mother more or less gave up her life to take care of me and my uncle. Watching him go through cancer was devastating for all of us. I was very close to my uncle. We would laugh and I found that there was no one who understood my journey more than someone else in my own home going through the same thing I was. Adversity can bond you with someone in a great way. I will never forget him and his legacy lives on forever. If you're not thinking of others throughout your journey here on earth, what is it all for?

If I had to speak in front of high school students or if I were to give a TED talk, I would speak about overcoming the odds. I have been through so many things in this journey and the most important lesson I've learned is that you have to believe in yourself and believe that you can do anything in spite of what's in front of you. I have faced death so many times and I learned along the way that you just have to bear down and get through it because you can. I think about the times I've been in the boxing ring when I faced golden glove champs and even pros and they were so much better than me. But I believe in myself because of the confidence of beating cancer and quite a few times when facing opponents better than me, I would win. I would tell myself over and over I can do this. It sounds stupid but it eventually started clicking in my head and I would surprise myself about how well I did. I've beaten cancer five times over a 12-year battle with cancer. I should have been dead a long time ago but I never gave up.

Every day, I would plan how I would win and no matter how tired I was I would plan how I would beat this day and win. Every obstacle is a challenge and I would never believe I could accomplish all the things I have but I did. Beating cancer is one of the toughest things anyone can do because of the everyday struggle. If, when I was first diagnosed, I had been told how many times my cancer would recur, I would never have believed I could have survived. But the thing is, anything can happen no matter what the situation and I know I keep saying it but believing in yourself is the key to overcoming anything and it all starts with you! What's your why?

My main reason for writing this book is to give back to others. I've had close to 1,000 hours of chemotherapy, over 100 units of radiation, and dozens and dozens of biopsies, along with two stem-cell transplants over the course of eight-and-a-half years. I lost weight, I lost my strength, and I lost joy. There were days that I just wanted to give up. But I didn't. Why?

You can call it divine intervention or just plain stubbornness, but I know it's a combination of both.

Getting back to training—and back into the boxing ring—helped me to feel alive again and I even got my brother, Vincent, involved. We didn't just train together, but Vincent also stepped up into the caregiver role when I needed it.

We have been interviewed by many different media, but SurvivorNet interviewed us and it was a family affair. We have been all-in through this journey. "We're all very close," Vincent told them. "I tried to be there as much as I could."

My mom went to appointments to ask questions, helped me schedule treatments, took notes, the whole nine yards. In all of it I realized the importance of being your own advocate. There's nothing glamorous about cancer but there is something glamorous about persistence and having the fortitude to fight. Having your family there for you through the cancer journey really does make a world of difference.

How can you give back in the face of adversity? I think the best advice I could give is just to be you. Each one of us has a calling from God on this earth. I've done lots of interviews and lots of media and none of that matters. All that matters is my own calling to give back. What is yours? It might be very different.

Chapter 7

NOTHING IN LIFE COMES EASY

"Failure isn't being knocked down. Failure is not getting back up."

My mission is to encourage others to fight instead of giving up. It's always too early to quit. I had to draw on deep reservoirs of strength and endurance to survive for years when I was told there was no cure for me. Throughout this time, the battle to fight negative thoughts has been the most difficult fight of all. But I never allowed myself to give in to those thoughts. My message is clear: make the decision to never ever give up, despite your circumstances.

My family has played a huge role in my strength. Every time I wanted to quit, or give up, they were right there and I just couldn't do it. That was something I think everyone needs, something to hold on to, to get them through the hardest times. And that's what my family did for me. They never quit on me and I didn't quit on them.

My hope is that this book will provide hope, strength, and inspiration to not only those battling cancer, but to those that are simply struggling in their daily lives for any reason. Even before I had cancer, I still had problems and I had to overcome them. Cancer was just the hardest one. I've been a fighter my whole life. So I hope my story will show others how to improve their lives in a positive way, and will give them strength to keep on going. I want to inspire people, in spite of their struggles, to chase after their dreams and goals, whatever they may be.

I have a lot of dreams, a lot of aspirations. I've always wanted a lot since I was a little kid, and each day I come closer and closer to achieving all of those things. I've accomplished much of what I've wanted to accomplish, even while fighting a deadly disease. I will be fighting cancer for the rest of my life because there is no cure and that's fine. I have learned to live with it. I've learned to embrace it. It's just, these are the things that I want and there's things that I fight for. The one thing I want to do most with my life is to change as many other lives for the good as humanly possible.

I always wanted to compete in something, but I just couldn't find what it was. So, after my first stem cell transplant, in which I lost 50% of my lung functioning, I started going to a boxing gym. The first time I walked in, I saw these two massive men that were fighting. And I was like, "Oh my God, this is for me. I got to do this." I had no hair, no strength, no nothing. I was puffy. I looked awful. I approached three coaches but no one would take me on because they were protecting me. But I finally found a coach who gave me a chance, and he said I had potential. I'm grateful to my boxing coach as much as I am to the doctors who have saved me.

When my boxing coach took me on it infused my brain with confidence and strengthened me even more! It gave me a lot of inner strength. And it was something that helped me better my mindset because when you fight, you get to see what kind of man you are that day.

Winning isn't everything but training is. It really wasn't about winning or losing, even though I hated losing—it was that I wanted to survive the rounds. Fighting made me feel as though I wasn't going to die, because how can someone who survives getting punched hundreds of times be at death's door?

Fighting in the boxing ring filled me with the hope that I would live. That was remarkable because my fear disappeared. "I'm too healthy to die," I thought. My mindset shifted from hospitals, negative words, treatments, and fear to empowering thoughts such as: "I'm doing too much! I'm doing too much to die. Cancer patients don't usually fight in a boxing ring!"

It taught me also that there's no excuses. It doesn't matter if you're sick or not. It taught me how to grind. It taught me how to deal with things like panic attacks. While I was fighting, I would get panic attacks. I had to learn how to deal with that and it helped me deal with everything else I'm facing today. It made me look forward to something because I couldn't really be around people. I always had a girlfriend, but I really didn't go out, and my twenties were literally taken away. So, I always looked forward to going to the gym and training with my partners and sparring and fighting. It's something that was all mine. And I think everybody needs to have something in their lives that drives them.

Fighting was something that taught me how to be strong while being sick, and going to the gym taught me how to be able to do things while I'm sick. The alternative was to stay on the couch or in bed and let my muscles atrophy. Getting out to the gym despite the immune system risk was what sustained me and gave me a better quality of life!

From there, I learned to have a life. I can take a nap at home and feel rotten for whole weeks at a time but I know I'm still a fighter. I can go out and do this, this, and this and in my mind it's an accomplishment and a win. This kind of thinking has helped me navigate. I can have a life because, well, the girls I've dated in the past needed to go do everything, and I went with them. When you have a physical illness, the primary issue is feeling as if you're left out, because you have friends doing other things you can't go and do.

When I was younger, I often felt like I was left out because everybody had a college experience, and mine was being sick. And then the people out of college traveled and did this and did that, but I was in a hospital bed. So, my thing was, I got to fight. I fought in the boxing ring and I fought in the hospital. I always want to win because that's my competitive nature. In the boxing ring I only got dropped once and that's it. But in the hospital, I always won. No matter if I got pneumonia, no matter what happened to put me in the hospital, I always got out again; I was always victorious. It was the fighting attitude that gave me a lot of confidence in myself and my life. And it's something that I'll do for the rest of my life as long as I can because it taught me how to be strong in different ways. Not just someone coming at you, because you got to beat the person up. It helped me get strong and to understand that the most important aspect that controls your entire life is your brain. This controls everything. Your mindset is everything. If there's a gift that cancer gave me it's that it made me into someone that I'm very proud of today. I'm very strong. And I wasn't like that growing up. I wasn't. But I am now.

The adversity I have faced is not a minor adversity. I relied ultimately on my mindset to rebuild the physical aspect or confidence aspect in order to rebuild the fighter aspect.

From the moment we first trained together, my trainer was like family to me. We didn't talk every day, but he'll always be family to me. He protected me. He acted like a parent, and he acted like a best friend. He taught me something that I loved, how to box. He helped me overcome the challenges in my head and heart. I kept losing a lot. I couldn't breathe. I would think, "How do I win if I can't breathe?"

But my coach wanted to teach me how to keep fighting as a boxer, because he wanted me to learn to keep fighting the cancer. He said to me, "I think I'm helping you find your own fight by letting you fight here because of the joy that it brings you. And that it teaches you that if you can win here, you can win there." And I'll never forget when he said that. Some moments stay with you forever, and I want to stop right now and speak to you the reader directly, and tell you: No matter what you're going through, please don't give up. You've got to make a plan to get busy doing something that you love - whatever that may be! Find your hobby that gives you a moment of joy and everlasting confidence. Find it and develop a routine. Whether it's hiking, walking, writing, working out at the gym, attending a Pilates class, serving the homeless, or any other thing. Keep searching until you find that one thing that gives you joy.

Once I started boxing with my new mentor, it all kind of just rolled into place. He had to be crazy for bringing a cancer patient who looked like he had no strength into the gym to train, but he did it and I will love him forever for it.

He was an amazing gift. While he taught me how to box in the ring, he taught me how to fight in all areas of my life. The boxing ring became the place I could compete and win, and that attitude carried over into all areas of my life. When you find yourself, you get this confidence that allows you to do things that you would not normally do and you take chances and try new things. Miracles happen every day!

But when you quit, it's all over. You must keep at it. You can't not do it.

Chapter 8

I SURVIVED THE PANDEMIC

"I've learned how to not be afraid. The first step to not being afraid is you first have to act like you aren't afraid and during that process your mind, body, and soul follow."

The Covid-19 pandemic was a very scary thing. Millions of people died and everyone's life was changed. People lost their jobs, lost family members, and lost their livelihood. Restaurants closed, businesses folded, and schools closed too as cities and states began scrambling to stop the loss of life.

It's very odd to be fighting for your life as the Lone Ranger, the young guy with cancer, and then be suddenly thrust into a world where everyone around you is fighting a virus. I was lucky enough that my family didn't lose their jobs and none of us got Covid.

When the outbreak happened, my doctor made it very clear how serious Covid was. He told me that because I've battled cancer for over a decade, I was high risk because I'm immune-compromised. It was scary but it was at least battling another thing like cancer.

When Covid started, I was working on projects I had wanted to work on for year, but suddenly everything was put on hold. Some things are still on hold to this day. Healthwise, I'm doing amazing, but I don't know if I'll start getting really sick or not. So, even though I'm so close to accomplishing my dreams, I have to wait till things get better because of how serious Covid is. I am very blessed that only one of my family members got Covid and he went through it well. I know many people, including friends, who had the virus and that was scary. The feeling I had when I was diagnosed with cancer again was almost the same feeling I had when Covid first happened. I felt that because I've been through hell with cancer for so many years, I was prepared for Covid and whatever curve balls were coming because of it. Last year I started planning for work. I had a book coming out, I was having a huge event for my Foundation, and I had partnerships for very big charities. Everything I wanted was right there but it had to be put on hold because of a new cancer diagnosis and staggering symptoms which needed addressing.

Now I didn't complain about it by any means because people lost their jobs, family members, and so many horrible things. Every time I went out, I always had a mask on, always washed my hands, and followed the protocol that was told to everyone. What stressed me out the most was that I don't know what's going to happen to me and I still had much I wanted to accomplish, no matter how long or short my life will be. Then last year I woke up one day and couldn't breathe right. I felt as though I had Covid and I truly felt when I was in the hospital I was going to die. Once they did the tests, I was lucky enough not to have Covid but instead I had pneumonia for the fourth time.

One night in the hospital, with my mom sleeping in the chair nearby, I laid in the bed shaking for hours. I finally got up and, with my oxygen mask on, I went into the bathroom and wrote 33 goodbye letters to the people I'm closest to.

They didn't know what kind of pneumonia I had so I had to have a biopsy of my lungs. Once they got the results, I was put on steroids and things got a lot better. But when I left the hospital, I still couldn't breathe right and this impacted my mindset and made me fearful. I couldn't go up a half flight of stairs.

So, every day, I trained like I was fighting for my life in case that day comes that I get diagnosed with Covid. Every time I turned on the TV, people were talking about Covid, work on a vaccine, and how many people had passed away. I trained and I trained some more because of how serious this thing was. I was very blessed that nobody I'm close with—friends or family— passed away from Covid. Then at the beginning of 2021 we were told that vaccines were available, and that took some stress off, but I was still nervous. To this day every time I leave the house, I have a mask on and hand sanitizer to clean my hands.

I didn't go on a lot of dates when all of this happened because I didn't want to get sick. The worst part about it was people couldn't live the way they did before the pandemic. I've been fighting for my life for 12 years so I know how to deal with the "what if's" and the fear. At the beginning of Covid I didn't leave my house just because so many people were dying and the people at highest risk were people like me that are immune-compromised.

But then I started going out more while still taking safety precautions, and eventually that fear went away. I told myself, "I'm going to take all the necessary steps to make sure I don't get it, but I choose to live my life." I hung out with friends and went on dates. During the day I would do work whether it was my job, training, or helping out my family because my grandparents moved in with us. I could tell that they were scared because of their age they are at high risk. But just like my story with cancer now I chose to live my life and do what I want within reason. And I tell people all the time that as long as you do what you got to do to stay safe go out and live your life!

After I got the first shot, I wasn't sick and then I had to wait a month to get the second one. So many people I know got so horribly sick from the second shot, including my family members, and I'm not going to lie I was nervous because I had chemo a couple days before the second one. I asked my doctor why I didn't get sick from either of the shots, and she said it's because I'm strong - and that made me feel good.

A positive mindset and encouraging words can strengthen you! All those years of being told my body is weak and blah-blah-blah—but guess what? It's stronger than ever! My life now is awesome. Work is picking up and I'm getting a lot of opportunities which makes me happy. Most importantly I live every day like it's my last, because Covid along with the cancer reminded me that life is too short. Fight the fear and be fearless with your own life and do what you want that makes you happy. Covid was that reminder for me and I'm happier than ever. In case anybody wants to know, I always wear a mask when I leave the house; I don't go to parties or over to people's houses that haven't been vaccinated. Yes, I live and do what I want but I stay smart and I'm ready more than ever to have a hell of a life like we all should.

At first, I was very nervous about the pandemic because so many people were getting sick and dying left and right. I didn't know what to think. Before it was all happening, I was preparing for my first major event for my Foundation where I was going to raise thousands of dollars which I would use to help families or people that are sick. Then next thing I knew, this outbreak happened and everyone was freaking out. During this time, I'm still getting chemotherapy and the way hospitals are they barely would let my mom came in and for the first time both my parents couldn't come in the room with me and that felt weird to me. That's when it really hit me. It wasn't the event not happening. It was looking at the room during chemo and not seeing my dad there that really affected me. It's weird how some things hit you but that's when it hit me that this is a very scary and serious thing. I started leaving the house more after I got the vaccine. But all and all, I am very lucky not to have gotten Covid. Like I tell people, if you follow the steps, you have a good shot at being okay and healthy. I don't know if I would have survived Covid, even though I survived cancer so many times. I'm just glad I was never in the situation to find out.

I'm very lucky I never got sick but just like my battle with cancer I had to battle Covid by not getting it. I'm a fighter and always will be. As I wrote this book I was in a constant battle. I chose to fight every step of the way, and just being able to capture these thoughts is empowering.

Since I was 22, I had a dream and it's something that I always felt in my heart I would do. I pictured myself writing books, one about my life and cancer journey, and the others perhaps about how I was able to get through the toughest times in my life when I thought I was going to die, or missing out on doing things, being depressed, wanting to give up, and all sorts of things. I always pictured myself going around the country or world giving speeches about my journey and about how I overcame so many obstacles, not just cancer but in my life in general.

During this time, I would have my own Foundation and I would be able to raise thousands of dollars to help families pay for treatments or drugs. I dreamed about having fundraisers to give money to cancer research or even just to help out families. My point is, I thought of all those things but every time I thought I would be able to do them, I would end up being really sick again. And this happened over and over and over again. And to be honest, there were times—well, actually quite a few times—I thought it was just a dream because there was no way I was going to survive. I mean, for example, I would go to bed so many nights not knowing if I would wake up. I would say my prayers asking God for strength and just another day to be alive. At the same time, there was something inside of me that thought God put me in this situation so I could overcome it and help people.

I have been able to achieve the dreams of giving global virtual interviews, as I talk about my journey. Since the pandemic has reduced travel, this isn't foreign now and it's the way the world works. Speakers do virtual speeches. Companies hold meetings virtually on Zoom.

Now through all the times I beat cancer I was helping people. I was doing all these interviews and I would do all these speeches and the more people I would inspire the more I thought this was why God put me on this earth. It wasn't to be an athlete; it was to be a picture of strength and of overcoming anything. But what would happen is I would get cancer again and I would get sicker and sicker and sicker. Since I was 23, I've been inspiring people and when I would beat cancer yet again, I had more confidence than ever that God made me go through this for that dream I had. So, while I was battling, I would tell myself, "You got to keep pushing, you can't give up, you can do something great, you got to hold on and move forward."

No matter how much I was suffering I couldn't give up, not just for my family and people who cared about me but for the people out there I could really help. The one time I really questioned whether I was going to make it was when I had brain cancer. My entire brain was filled with cancer and I had 47 other areas in my body with cancer. When I found out I went into remission, I knew I could do anything and God gave me a gift by giving me a miracle. I went from almost not making it to being cancer free. And that whole year I took care of myself and trained strongman training.

At the same time I was trying to find a writer to do my book because that was always the first step. But that year I couldn't find the right one. So, a couple days after the new year, a year after my miracle happened, I was on the phone with my manager and she asked me what she could do for me. I told her I would really like to have a book about my life so I could travel and speak about my story.

My manager put me in touch with an amazingly successful woman whose name is Tammy Kling . She had written many books and was so good at creating bestsellers, but she was very authentic. I could feel her heart to help others. Nothing felt more right than to have her guide me in writing my book.

And after that call my manager began setting up an event for my Foundation in which we were planning to raise tens of thousands of dollars if not hundreds of thousands of dollars. And I knew while the book was being written I would have this event and from the amount

I raised I could do all the things I was thinking about for years. Then the Covid outbreak happened.

If the event had been planned for just two weeks earlier, we would have been able to hold it. But we had to wait. I didn't complain because it wasn't just me who was suffering. So many people lost their jobs or lost loved ones during the pandemic and I was so confused by it all. I would say I wasn't as afraid as some people were because I faced death so many times. But I was mad because at the time, unlike other years, I was so strong and so healthy. I could do anything. I could travel, I could make speeches; I could do anything and I had been waiting to be in this position for almost a decade but yet again I had to wait. It wasn't the fear of the pandemic, it was more so I had to wait again. Except the difference is I was always sick so I had to focus on that but this time even though I'm still doing treatments I had to change my mindset and try to be as productive as possible.

In spite of not being able to do everything I wanted to do, I was still able to help people who reached out to me, whether a friend or someone who reached out online. Most people over the years reach out because they want help with battling cancer. But this time I was helping people deal with the fear of this virus that was killing so many people. I was familiar with this fear because of almost dying all those times. So, I was trying to help people calm down and make them realize if they follow the precautions, they will be okay. So yes, I wasn't doing everything that was planned and I was upset about it. But the reality is I was still making a difference. Yes, it wasn't as big of a difference as I planned on doing but it was still something. After the first few months I wasn't afraid anymore I was just trying to learn to be patient. Anyone who knows me will tell you being patient is something I'm horrible at. I just want to do do do do and for the first time I wasn't sick like I had been, so I had to learn how to be patient in the job world which is something I've gotten a lot better at.

I'm choosing to look at this horrible situation as a time to learn from my big weakness—not being patient—and I tried to be as productive as possible. I've remained positive because I know how important that is. Learning to be positive and patient has made me a stronger person. I'm more patient with people and I think that's made me a better person, so for that I'm grateful. I stopped being mad about waiting because it wasn't doing me any good.

While I wasn't working, I tried to be as healthy as possible. Now during this time, my resting heart rate was 137. So, I started boxing again during the pandemic and with the help of an elevation mask my resting heart rate is 73. So, during the pandemic I made it my goal to be as healthy as humanly possible. Yes, I was afraid because I really thought I was going to die during this pandemic when I was in the hospital. But my breathing got better than it ever had in my entire life.

While I was in the hospital with pneumonia, I had to deal with fighting for my life again and that was the worst time of the whole pandemic. But I'm blessed because I'm doing what I love again which is working out, and writing a book too, and I'm healthier than ever. So yes, I didn't get Covid but I got something that was very bad and it made me think. After I beat brain cancer my goal was to be as big and strong as humanly possible. But now I'm still very strong but it's about being as healthy as possible. There's one thing money can't buy and that's health.

One thought I want to share with whoever I'm talking to is that this pandemic should make us realize how important our health is and we should take the best care of ourselves no matter what.

When I do my interviews and give speeches, I will say what I learned—which I knew before but it's just glaringly more important now! Your health and mine is critical to life. Each one of us should take the best care of ourselves possible. I'm glad I got sick because my focus was really wrong before that. I just hope that whoever is reading this that you start taking care of yourself. You owe it to yourself to take care of yourself. All the years I was sick I always felt bad and it sucks. This pandemic should be a reminder to stay strong and healthy because when the time comes that, God forbid, you get sick, you need to give yourself the best chance at beating it. Now will we all die one day? Yes, of course. But let's not die before our time and no matter how old we are, it's a reminder to live our God-given purpose. All that training that I did all those years helped me beat cancer for years. It was not for nothing! It made me strong mentally and physically.

Chapter 9

IN HER OWN WORDS

"You're the definition of strength. You have been there through the good, the bad, and the ugly. You are relentlessly fierce when it comes to the people you love. You're my best friend."

During the writing of this book my writing coach urged me to include words from my family, to help them give their side of the story. I agreed wholeheartedly because my journey has been nothing without them in it as a major part of my life. My family is my life, and since writing this is so therapeutic, I'm hoping it helps them to contribute to my story here too. Mom, you deserved your one chapter, for all that you've done and been to me. I love you!

IN MOM'S OWN WORDS:

Being told that your child has a potentially lethal disease is something that you never think is going to happen to you. It's something that takes your life and it freezes you and all you think about is, "What can I do to make him well? How can I make his life better?" You really find out who you are when something like this happens.

Even at this present time, thank God, Anthony is stable but in the back of your mind you think, "What would be the next step if his situation becomes unstable again?" I have gone from daily research to a state of maintenance with my son, myself and our family around us. Anthony and I in particular have been through all of it together every moment. There are times that I wasn't allowed to go in with him for the scans, for reasons such a Covid, but those are the only times that we have been separated through this. We have a connection, a bond, a camaraderie that doesn't come along every day that is very special to both of us.

Not to say that I don't have a special bond with my other two boys, because I do. But with Anthony it's different because we have been to the edge of the cliff looking down together, but we never ever stopped trying and hoping. It has been and will continue to be a very emotional journey for both of us because when you're dealing with that six-letter word, the stress and fear play with you on a daily basis. One day you're good and the next day it can be gone because your child can start showing side effects from the six-letter word or the present treatment and your job is never to stop. You are never in an off position. I've learned things about Anthony that I was not aware of and he has learned things about me. You never really completely know someone but if you go through something like this together you begin to have a good handle on who they are. When you watch somebody endure what I've watched my son endure, you know them very well.

At times I feel guilty when I have a day in which I feel very energetic and my physical being feels good for my age. I feel guilty because I know my son still has aches and pains and residual pain from all the treatments. My feelings of guilt come into play when he's not having a great day and I played a role in those treatments that he went through. I always tried to play a role in whatever treatment was chosen because when it's for your child you never trust anybody or any doctor completely. I never have and I never will. I have to have a say in Anthony's treatment because it's for my child and his well-being. I always did my own research. I took that and combined it with what was suggested by the oncologist. I took what I researched and combined it with what the oncologist suggested and then the next treatment would be decided together between us and the oncologist.

There were times when Anthony would say to me, "I don't have a good feeling about this, Mom. I don't think I'm going to get through it." And I would always be positive and say, "This is the best thing now that we can try and you will get through it because you will not go on my watch." I always said that to him, "You will not go on my watch," meaning, "If I'm there you're not leaving this world." There were many moments when Anthony said, "Maybe this is it, Mom, there are no other treatments." But I always got together with the oncologist and we always found something for Anthony, whether it be a trial or another FDA-approved drug.

Whatever the treatment was, we chose it because it was the best option at that time. You're always searching for treatments or for a resolution to this spiraling nightmare that you're in together. I do have to say that it was not always peaches and cream being together. Some of the hospital rooms were very small and because of his low counts he was not able to leave the room so we would be there together every minute of every hour of every day! Sometimes that could be a challenge! But at the end of each trial, we remained close and tight because when you go through something like this with someone else there's no other way you can make it but to be tight and close to each other.

What has it taught me about life and adversity?

The day I was told that my son had lymphoma, everything stopped. Life as I knew it was gone, and I didn't know whether it would ever be the same again. We have a close-knit family and life became very complicated, life became very hectic, and life became one big roller coaster within the world of cancer. We have always tried to enjoy the good times and to appreciate good news whenever it comes our way, but in the back of all of our minds has always been the thought, "Is this cancer ever going to go away and leave Anthony and our family alone?"

You can't trust what's going on in your life at any given time because it changes with the snap of a finger. Each day is different and your life is different. When things change in your life to such a drastic measure as being diagnosed with cancer you realize that you don't have control over anything. Sometimes life simply unravels. When something like this happens to a loved one, you truly discover what type of person you are and what type of people you are surrounded by. In the world of cancer, I have learned to be a very take-charge, full-steam-ahead, don't-take-no-for-an-answer type of person. You have to be that way with cancer because the alternative is unbearable.

I don't think about losing my son because that's not an option. You do everything you need to do each day to give your loved one a quality of life. Even when your loved one is very sick and very weak and, in their eyes, they are telling you they're done because they can't take it anymore, you have to be the strength for your loved one and then they rise up again. Their lives within this world of cancer change constantly and you have to let them know that they are loved and that you are fighting right along with them; it's not just their fight alone. It's the fight of the family and together we are winning and we will continue to win because our loved one is strong and he will survive.

Love,

Mom

Chapter 10

STEVEN

"He was our shining light."

My uncle Steven was a beautiful person inside and out. He was also an incredible artist, an actor, and he worked so well with his hands in carpentry too. My uncle was multi-talented and he could've done anything with his hands that he put his mind to. If someone asked him to do something in the way of carpentry, he could make his hands do it! My uncle was a very bright and compassionate person and he was just a great guy. He meant so much to me right up to the day he died. We shared a lot in that final year together as we both fought a common enemy.

When my uncle was healthy, he was a great actor. He started acting in high school plays and went on to do more acting in college. He also took acting lessons in New York City and he did a couple of commercials and some short films and he was active in community theater. He also wrote plays and directed. While doing all of this, he started his own business called Peanut Butter Classics and he made his own peanut butter and put different flavors in it, which was very creative!

Renaissance man was the best description of him because he just wanted to do everything. He wanted to try and to experience everything in life and he pretty much did.

I asked my grandmother how he was when he was an infant and she said that of all her five children he was by far the calmest and he slept all the time, for which was she was thankful!

It seems he'd been perfect even then because he was well behaved and he entertained his younger siblings with all different games that he played. One Christmas he asked Santa Claus for a magician's kit, and after he opened it he entertained the family most of the day with his different tricks. Even as a kid, he was entertaining and funny and just so clever.

School did not interest him much because intellectually he was just so ahead of his years, but he got through it with average grades. He could've done much better because he was so clever but he was perpetually bored as a student, even though he was popular.

He did not like sports like his brother and sister. Uncle Steven preferred acting and writing and he had a heart of an artist. People always said he was a great dresser. After he passed away, a woman told me a memory she had of him from when they were just kids. He was new to the school because the family had moved, and on the first morning of classes he came in wearing a shirt and tie and a sports jacket, and he was only in third grade! She never forgot that.

He loved to dress up and he didn't have to go to fancy stores to shop because he had a great sense of style. He would go to consignment shops and buy clothes there and he had a body where his clothes fit well on him. He could wear anything and he just looked great anytime he went out. He was a big giver too. He loved shopping and he loved buying gifts for people, and always managed to get the best gifts that fit the personality of the person he was giving to.

Throughout his life Uncle Steven always wanted to help, and I remember that he always rooted for the underdog. He just loved to help people whether they were old or young or in between. He helped anybody who needed help and he gave a lot of advice to young people and helped them through the hard times in school as well. People could always count on Steven to give them good advice and always be there for them.

Dating life for Steven when he was younger was a little difficult, and he wasn't as successful in that department especially in middle school or high school. Even though he was so well liked, he told me that he became friends with a lot of the women even if they didn't necessarily want to be in a more romantic relationship with him. In college, he started really dating and getting to know a lot of people. He never married but he had quite a few serious relationships. Regardless of what happened in those relationships, he was always there for his friends and he never burned the bridge.

Upon graduating from college, he went to work with his father in the machine shop. He did quite well and enjoyed it but he would always have to do something on the side. For instance, he might take a car apart and put it back together even better than before because he just loved doing things like that. Upon leaving the machine shop he went into carpentry and he continued with his peanut butter and also with his acting which was his first love!

QUOTES

1) "Even if you live in a cave, a leaf blows in once in a while."
2) "Even when we are launching bombs at each other—how peaceful things look from space!"

Uncle Steve cared about people. He tried to help everyone. He spent a lot of time with young people, listening to their problems and offering advice. He helped the elderly by doing things around the house for them, shopping for them, having dinner with them. They loved him and he returned their love. When he passed, a man who came to the wake said he would call Steve and ask him to do odd jobs around the house. This man had three little girls, and when the girls heard

Steve was coming, they would jump for joy and say, "Steve is coming! Hooray!" This man said that whenever Steve came to the house, he always played games with the girls before doing his work.

At Uncle Steve's funeral, a man came up to me and was crying with tears rolling down his cheeks. He said, "Why did someone like Steve have to leave us who was such a great person?" And one woman told me all people should be like Steve. What a wonderful world this would be.

Steven before his diagnosis:

- He had trouble swallowing.
- He had a constant hiccup.
- He would get night sweats.
- Throat would be itchy and something always felt was in his throat.
- Would get fevers consistently.

After his diagnosis, we had a lot of talks as we both fought cancer together while living under the same roof.

Chapter 11

FAMILY

"Family is not an important thing; it is everything." - Michael J. Fox

My family means everything to me. My parents, my brothers, my grandparents, my uncles, aunts, and cousins. I would do anything for each and every one of them, no matter what. Now I may have a crazy Italian family, but they are the reason why I fought so hard. I not only fought to survive so they wouldn't be hurt but I also fought so hard so that they would be proud of me. To be honest, all I've ever wanted my entire life is to do something that makes them proud of me.

My mom is the strongest person I've ever met in my entire life. She is always there for her kids and she will fight like hell for them whenever she needs to. There's no person on the planet my mom would back down from when it is about her children. My brothers and I are her entire world. Now we may not have had the most money growing up but my brothers and I got everything we've ever wanted. Most importantly, no matter the mistakes we may have made, no matter the situation we may be in, she will always be there to listen to us and offer counsel and advice. And even though we may not like what she has to say, she's always right. That's why when I get bad news or something happens to me health-wise, I don't listen to my doctors first. I listen to my mom first and, the weirdest thing is, she never went to medical school but she is always right. If she thinks my cancer got worse, she's right. If she thinks my scan is going to be good, she's right. If I'm dating a girl, she'll tell me if she's the right one for me; even if I love the girl dearly, Mom will tell me the truth because she has always been right.

Now there were times where I was so mad at my mom when I was sick. She was so hard on me at times that I was resentful. But over the years I've become grateful for what she and my dad did. By not coddling me and by being hard on me, they gave me the opportunity to be strong. And because I've gotten so strong it's hard to be mad at them. I don't just look up to my mom and think she's the strongest woman in the world, but she is also my best friend, and I would go to the ends of the earth to make her happy.

I am blessed to have an amazing family!

From the time I was a little boy all I wanted to do is grow up and be my dad. When kids are young, they may want to be like a movie star, or a professional athlete, or whatever it may be. I never wanted to be like any of them. All I wanted is to be like my dad. He also has given me and my brothers everything we've ever wanted in our lives. I played hockey because that was Dad's favorite sport and he'd played it as well. I got into the school he went to for college and my plan before I got sick was to join the ROTC program there. If for some reason I wasn't going to be a professional hockey player, I was going to join the army with the hope of becoming an army ranger just like my dad. From what I can remember, Dad said he was proud of me only three times my entire life. Now some people can say that's messed up, but I prefer it that way. The reason is when I hear Dad says he's proud of me, it means I did something great. Whether it was an accomplishment or I did something that helped a bunch of people, it means something to me.

My parents have pushed me and my brothers to be the best versions of ourselves possible. They support all of our dreams and will do anything to help us get to that. I just don't think you can get better parents than I have. They've made us so strong and taught us that there are no excuses, just results, and that has pushed us to do great things.

Both my parents have been to every doctor's appointment I've ever had during my years with cancer. Just take a moment to think about that. My parents have important jobs and two other children and they found ways to always be there for me. For the past two years I've been asking them to let me do it on my own but they just don't want me to be alone. It's very sweet, to be honest. In my room I have a bed, a nice TV, and a couch. The first couple years I was battling cancer my dad slept on that couch every single night. And over the years if I was very sick, Dad would stay in my room with me. Not because I asked that of him but that's what he wanted to do. He'd work 16-hour days because he's a vice president at PepsiCo, and instead of lying in a comfortable bed to sleep at night, he chose the couch. He doesn't know this but I can't tell you how grateful I am to have that kind of support. Nowadays I sleep alone because I'm very strong and I know how to deal with things now. But I'll never forget all the nights I was throwing up, or how many times he changed my sheets and he and my mom would clean my bed for obvious reasons. I'm not going to explain why but I'm sure you can understand why they would do that.

I think another reason why I'm still alive was because of how much my parents pushed me. They were always hard on me in my weakest moments. At the time I would be so mad, but looking back on it, it really helped me be very strong. My mom, on top of having a job and running a household, always got me the best appointments at the best times at the best hospital. If I needed something, she got it—whether it was medicine or something else. Thinking about it right now my mom is literally superwoman. She's always doing something and always getting the job done. I tell everyone that if it weren't for my parents, I wouldn't be alive. Too many things have happened and doing it on my own would just be impossible. We are talking about 12 years of so many ups and downs and I am forever grateful for everything they have done for me. And because of all of that I want to give them the world. That's why I'm working so hard not just to help people all around the world, but also to support my parents because they deserve it more than anyone.

Now my parents aren't the only people I'm going to talk about. My brothers played a big role in my journey as well. My brother Vincent moved out to California to chase his dream to be an actor. Let me tell you, he is very good. I mean, he is amazing at his craft. And yet, after my second transplant, Vincent stopped chasing his dream to help out with me. And speaking of brothers, it was my youngest brother Michael who gave his cells for my transplant. Funny story about that—I used to make fun of Michael for having red hair and honestly, it's not even red. But before my transplant my beard, when it grew out, was brown and blond. Since the transplant, my beard grows red now and I think it's because of the cells Michael gave me! Talk about karma. Mom and I also believe that even though the transplant didn't cure me, it changed my body by making it stronger, and now chemotherapy works better than it did before I got his cells. Anyway getting back to Vincent ... Dad had to go back east to work so Vincent took his place in so many ways. When I would be in the bathroom for hours passing clots out of my, well, you-know-what, he'd stay in the bathroom hearing me make awful noises because it was so painful. There was a time in the hospital that he was so tired from staying up with me, he opened his eyes and asked Mom and me why there was a parrot in the room. So much sleep deprivation made him see things that really weren't there. The point of me saying this is how much he is really helping. When I was in a wheelchair, he would push me. When I had to go to hyperbaric oxygen treatments for my bladder, he was there. He was with me for every blood transfusion, every biopsy, every doctor's appointment and he did that long after my transplant. And, Vincent, if you are reading this, thank you for your sacrifice; it meant more to me than you'll ever know. Thank you, bro, love ya.

My youngest brother Michael is also amazing and he's the one who gave me his cells. The gift of life. Every time I saw him, he would make me laugh and have a great time, no matter how sick I was or how bad any of it was. He's several years younger than me but I'm very close with him. He always would text me before chemo, scans, biopsies, and the list go on and he still does that to this day. Now he's very tough and doesn't show his emotions. He bottles them up. But I always felt so bad for how much I scared him by being sick. He never showed it but I knew it was going on. I would do anything for him because he's the kindest guy I've ever met. He did a very big thing by giving me his cells. That sacrifice meant the world to me. And even though we are blood brothers we are closer because he gave me his cells and he's part of me now and I love it.

My family means the absolute world to me. Everything I do in my life and everything I will do is to make them proud of me. No matter how many fights we get in or when we are mad at each other, we still love each other unconditionally. I was raised to always look after my brothers because I am the oldest. Now it was very hard to do that when I was so sick but I figured it out because it is important. A big reason why I never stop fighting and give up is so that they don't have to deal with the pain of losing me. I know from losing my uncle a couple years ago the damage that such a loss does to a family. And I refuse to let that happen and I will do whatever I have to do to make sure they don't feel that pain again. No matter how much I suffer I won't let them down. I promise you that much and I thank them and I thank God as well for making me so strong.

Chapter 12

CANCER IS A GIFT

"It's through my greatest battle that
I became the man I always wanted to be."

My biggest childhood dream was to be a hockey player and go pro if I could. When I was playing hockey in my youth, the greatest feeling I had was when I scored a goal. It was a better feeling than getting an A on a test I had studied weeks for. Even a better feeling than when I would ask a girl to be my girlfriend and she said yes. I could go on and on about how scoring a goal made me feel the best. After I broke my leg, I was searching to find something that gave me that feeling. At one point I told myself, "I guess that's it; I'm not going to feel that way again, but at least I got to experience the feeling in my life." I just let the hope of it returning fade. I left it in the past. But cancer gave me that feeling again because it gave me the opportunity to give back!

My first speech I made about my cancer was at a VFW (Veterans of Foreign Wars) meeting. I spoke three times at a VFW and the crowd was made up of people of all ages. For my first speech, which was a charity event, I brought a pair of my boxing gloves with me in case someone wanted to see them. Now obviously I know I'm not a professional boxer, but something told me, what the hell, just bring them. I spoke about how I was a boxer in hopes of showing people that you can do anything while battling cancer. After my speech, a couple took me aside and told me that their son had leukemia and they wondered if I would meet him. Of course, I said, yes absolutely. When I met their son, who was just five or six years old, he said to me, "Hi, Anthony, my name is Timmy and I have cancer just like you." So, I told him, "Yeah, buddy, don't worry; we are totally going to beat this thing." While I was talking to him, he kept staring at the gloves. He looked at his mom and said, "Mommy, I want to be a boxer like Anthony. Can I do it, Mommy? I really wanna do it!" That was the first time I realized I made a difference and that kid wanted to do what I did even though he was so sick. So, I gave the kid the gloves and you could tell he was so happy.

The feeling I got from this experience was something I've never felt before. When I was driving home, I called my girlfriend crying because I felt so good. I couldn't believe that someone would be inspired by me. It was at that moment I knew I had made a difference and also at that moment I knew what I wanted to do with the rest of my life: I want to help give hope, strength, and inspiration to anyone who needs it.

Hockey was my world and there are even days I still miss the feeling of skating on the ice. I felt so free and so relaxed. After I broke my leg, I couldn't even watch hockey on the television for years until after I met that young kid with leukemia and gave him my gloves. So many of my friends went on to play hockey in college and flourished at it, and some of them even made it to the pros. I was never jealous of them. I was very happy for them because hockey is one of the most competitive sports in the world, and being able to play NCAA is so difficult. All those players, for the most part, played on the best teams at a young age. I didn't start playing on the best teams till I was 17. I don't think it was because I wasn't good enough when I was younger; it just didn't work that way for me and that's okay. Every day, I would dream of the day I could finally say I made it as a hockey player. Still, the fact that I didn't make it is okay because it's not what God had planned for me. It's like the old saying, "Man plans, and God laughs." I asked God for strength and I got it, and I am forever grateful for it all because I didn't know that his plans were so much greater.

Over the years I've been given opportunities to speak and I would always get so nervous even though all I had to do was tell my story. It wasn't until I was asked to speak at the blood cancer gala that I stopped getting so nervous about public speaking and giving interviews. I had an entire room filled with celebrities, very successful businessmen, musicians, and executives. I was so nervous and spoke for about 15 minutes and it was one of the best feelings I've ever had. Every time I'm on stage or in front of the camera I have so much confidence and I know I help raise awareness and help others so it's all good on that end.

For a long time in my younger years, I felt like the world was against me and I couldn't find my niche in life. So many nights I would think about how to get that feeling back. How to do something that I will truly succeed in. Something that I know will make a difference. I remember once I was asked to speak at the middle school I attended when I was young. I always told myself those people who are asked to speak in front of all those children must do something impressive, so when I got asked, I was inclined to go. I got out of the car and got in my wheelchair and I remember all those kids looking at me. Now this was during the eight months that I've largely forgotten due to the treatment I was going through, so I really don't remember much of what I said. But my brother recorded my talk so I'm able to watch it and know I did a great job. I also received letters from the kids, and reading those letters really made me feel like I made a difference to the kids and I'm sure it motivated me to beat cancer.

For some reason a year ago, I was walking to my room and I remembered something from the day I spoke to the middle school students. One of the kids came up to me and thanked me for my speech and told me how it made him feel better because his dad had died from cancer. The great thing about speaking for the most part is that no matter how injured you are or how sick you are, you can most likely do the speech in almost any condition you are in and it will still inspire other people and make a difference in their lives.

When I'm up on the stage or in front of the virtual camera I feel so free just like I did when I was playing hockey. I get to tell people about my journey and hopefully help them through theirs. Telling my story is something I will do for the rest of my life. When you are speaking, you get to see the audience and you can feel it when you are affecting them in a positive way.

It's an amazing feeling and it's the same feeling I had when I scored a goal in hockey. For anyone who is reading this, you've got to keep pushing and trying to find the thing that makes you feel fulfilled. Feeling free, confident, happy and all of that is what it's all about. When you find that thing you love, embrace it, keep doing it, and work on getting better at it. I take videos of myself every week practicing my public speaking in order to get better at it. Just because I think I'm good at it doesn't mean I can't get better. I find my flaws and I discover ways to present something better. I do that so when the time comes and I'm asked to speak, I do an amazing job. If I do an amazing job, I'm helping people and that's what I want to do. I usually take videos of myself speaking in the middle of the night when everyone is asleep. I figure if I can do it when I'm half asleep and I do very well, then when I feel good, I'll do even better. I'm just so blessed that God drove me to the position to find something I love doing. It makes me so happy just thinking about it and I thank God for it all.

Another thing is no matter how sick I am if someone reaches out to me needing help, even if it's not about cancer, I am there. Over the years, so many people I don't even know have reached out to me and I'm happy to talk with them. I figure if they don't even know me and are reaching out, they must really be going through a hard time.

Not long ago, I became acquainted with a family whose five-year-old daughter was battling leukemia and she was screaming every second of the day. Unfortunately, they couldn't afford pain medicine for their daughter because their insurance didn't cover it. I had already been speaking with this family for months before the pain started and I really cared for them. The little girl was so sweet and the parents were amazing. I know what it's like to be in so much pain, so I would encourage the parents to take their daughter to the hospital. They did and she was given the drugs she needed to ease the pain. I sent the family some money so that they could afford the rest of the drugs I told them to get. Luckily, I was right and they were able to control the girl's pain, and she even ended up beating the cancer, so I'm so happy about that. Now, it's not like I sent them a thousand dollars, but I was able to help cover the cost so that the little girl had what she needed. I still talk to the family to this day and I'm so happy she's healthy and happy.

My point is that I don't like people suffering and if I can help in any way, I will figure out how to do it. Whether it's a phone call to someone battling depression, or someone wanting to get their faith back, I'm there. Unfortunately, I can't help everyone but if the opportunity arises, I am there no matter what. I am so blessed that I've learned so much and gotten so strong from my journey that I have the ability to help others. It makes me feel like this battle and all the suffering was worth it. I could go on and on about all the different conversations I've had with people of all ages. But I'm saying this because I'm passionate about making a difference while I'm still here. Whether it's inspiring a bunch of kids at school or helping a little girl get healthy so she can fulfill her dream of riding horses, that's what I live to do. I'm just so blessed that people think of me as someone they can turn to. I am always happy to get emails, messages on social media, or phone calls. If I can help, I will. Unfortunately, I haven't helped everyone I've spoken to but I'm trying my best to get better and better every day.

Chapter 13

THE SIDE EFFECTS OF CANCER SUCK

"There can only be one state of mind as you approach any profound test; total concentration, a spirit of togetherness, and strength."
- Pat Riley

I've been fortunate that my radiologist is one of the best in the world and has worked miracles for so many patients. Not only is he a great guy but he tells it like it is and always gets to the point. I remember my best friend got me tickets for a trip to the Cayman Islands with my brother, Michael; however, I had to have a scan right before we left. When I got the results, unfortunately it showed cancer in a dangerous spot.

So, we had to delay the trip while I underwent radiation therapy. Then I made a horrible decision going right after the two weeks of radiation. The thing is, every time I've gotten radiation, it has worked beautifully and it has never failed. I've had over 100 radiation treatments and I sat on that freezing table every single time. Almost every time before the radiation I would have to take pain meds because of the pain I was in. Every single time I had radiation therapy I had the first slot and woke up so early to beat New York City traffic. My radiation treatments typically lasted two to three weeks max, five days a week, and I had the weekends off. There was a time when I had cancer in my back and I was told by my doctor straight up, "Anthony, you have to do this as soon as possible because if you don't there's a good chance you won't be able to walk again." So obviously it was hard to take that in because the thought of not being able to walk scared the hell out of me.

Even in my situation now I have something in my back and in my right quad. Luckily when it popped up my cancer made it basically go away, but I still got my radiation tattoos in case whatever it is grows and I need the treatment. Getting radiation for me is very scary stuff. Being told you can be paralyzed, or that it might not work, and thinking of what will happen if this doesn't work, it's honestly very scary. You can be having such a great day but then the doctors tell you that you aren't doing well so you have to step up. During the treatments the only thing that happened was I would get dry skin. Sometimes my pain would be worse but the majority of the negatives is the dry skin and my counts get lower. So, there were times that my hemoglobin level was just barely normal even before treatment, so after the treatments were done it would drop a lot. As I've said before, when you have a low hemoglobin level you can be in the best shape of your life and yet simply going up a flight of stairs can be a problem. For the most part I haven't needed that many infusions from the radiation but it's happened.

The biggest problem I've had with radiation is what it does down the road. I had a 13-cm mass in my hip and because it was so big I was in great pain. I was on pain meds and using pain patches, so the doctors decided they needed to be aggressive in treating the mass. They made the dose of radiation higher than I've ever had, but the great thing was the mass went away and I wasn't in that much pain anymore and I didn't have a limp. Still, months later I woke up one day and the lower abdominal muscle felt like bone. I mean, think about a muscle feeling like bone. It's absolutely crazy to think about it. I'm getting physical therapy and for 20 to 30 minutes before PT, I get massages. I have a lot of scar tissue damage and the biggest problem is that every time I get radiation, I'm in pain. The radiation has caused a lot of nerve damage in several places of my body and that sucks. I have a limp that's getting better along with knee problems all because of the radiation treatments. When I'm told I need more radiation, I don't get upset over the fact that I have to go to the hospital every day. I get upset because every time I've gotten radiation, I've had permanent damage.

So honestly, I'd rather get chemotherapy than radiation because of the permanent damage it has caused. Now with chemotherapy the game is everything and anything can happen. Some chemotherapies I've gotten have only left me fatigued. Then there were times I had chemotherapy and afterward when I put clothes on, I felt like my skin was literally on fire. When I was in high school, I lit a cigar and got burned by the match—and after the chemo that same burning feeling was in my whole body.

The doctors can tell you what to look out for, so what I've learned is to get medicine in case something happens. For example, if there's a chance chemo might make me constipated, I asked for something to help with that. Every chemotherapy I've ever gotten has always made my skin itchy. To think about it, I've been itchy for about 12 years but that's something I've just had to get used to. But the positive of getting chemotherapy is it has taught me how to be mentally strong. It's taught me how to push myself when I'm so sick in every way you can possibly think of. It's made me believe in myself because it hasn't killed me, it just has made me stronger. I have to do chemotherapy or immunotherapy for the rest of my life. Some may say that's the most awful thing I've ever heard. I don't think that at all because of the benefits I've gotten from it. It's taught me how to fight adversity. It's taught me how to be grateful for every day I'm not sick.

Chemotherapy has humbled me and at the same time has given me so much confidence that I can get through everything. And the most important thing is it fights my cancer so I can have the most important thing—which is being alive. I choose to look at getting treatment like that as opposed to making it a death sentence. It's part of my life now just like taking vitamins is part of others' lives. It teaches me how to get the job done no matter how sick or how much pain I'm in.

When I'm sitting in the chair waiting to get chemo, the most frustrating thing is being stuck four to five times just to get the IV in. Sometimes I had to get chemo every week, sometimes every other week, sometimes every three weeks. Finally, I chose to take the double dose of treatment I'm on so I can only go to the hospital once a month! I mean, how incredible that is. I get to just go once a month and I am so blessed about that.

Nowadays I go much more often because I do physical therapy. My first week I couldn't walk with my right knee bent without falling. Now I can walk with my knee bent without a limp after a week because of how much I pushed myself. The physical therapists do amazing work and I'm so happy the right side of my body with the majority of the problems I have is getting better. I was told there was a chance I may not ever get better but I didn't get negative and get down on myself. I told myself I am going to get better! A week into it I was doing so much better and it was the same week I had treatment! So, my point is, even with my treatment I was training as a boxer, working, going to physical therapy, and most importantly, I have a life! For those people who say you can't have a life on treatment, that isn't true. Of course, cancer treatment has brought me to my knees at some points in my journey, but it also has uplifted me and made me a better man no matter what. So yes, it made me suffer a lot and I mean more than I could ever write down. But it also has made me a stronger, better person than I could ever write down on a piece of paper. I look at my cancer treatment as a gift, not as a sentence.

One of the things that's soothing for cancer patients and probably most humans battling anything, is an animal. Throughout my life I've always had a pet. My first pet was a rabbit and the whole family loved her until she passed away when I was a kid. I've had two rabbits, I had a cat, I have a dog named Zino who we've had for about six-and-a-half years. I also have a Yorkie named Bella; she weighs only about five pounds. It sounds so weird but I never understood how people could love their animals so much, as if it was a human being. But with Bella I think of her as my daughter. Yes, you can laugh at me all you want but that dog brings me so much joy I can't even explain it. When I was battling brain cancer my first memory of her was when I woke up and she was right next to my bed looking right at me. I remember telling myself, *Who is this little cute thing?* She was a little bigger than the palm of my hands. At that time, I was very, very sick. I was in a wheelchair, I was very thin and had no appetite and no energy. Even though my family was always present, I felt so alone. My girlfriend and I had broken up that year, even though I felt very close to her and was in love with her. The friends I talked to and hung out with stopped being friends with me. Whether it was because I was always in the hospital and sleeping all the time, to be honest, I don't know. Through my journey I've always had to bring myself back. I would lose all strength, energy, and everything else that goes along with that. Then I would beat cancer, get strong again, and get my life back again. It's a tough thing to deal with because every time you beat cancer, something is taken from you. Whether it's physical or mental. Something is always taken away. Little by little you start to lose yourself and that's a very hard thing to accept and deal with. You have to work your butt off to be able to get your entire life back and once I got it all back, my cancer would come back and the same cycle continued and continued. Even though I had my family I always felt lonely when I was really sick. It wasn't their fault at all; it's just that it's a battle only you can face. Just you and God. My parents work, my brother works or is at school and the same thing goes with my other brother. When I wasn't in a relationship there were a lot of times I felt truly lonely. I felt like there was nobody I could connect with to help with the loneliness. Feeling lonely is not feeling bad for yourself. You just feel lost, empty, and all those feelings come up. Then I would get to a point where I'd ask myself, *What's the point to all of this?* I would keep telling myself, *I'm going to be somebody and I'm going to change lives. I'm going to make a difference so people don't feel the way I have felt.*

Yes, I went to therapy a few times and to be honest it doesn't work for me. My current therapist is great and he helps me with my PTSD. But I'm at a great point in my life and I'm slowly becoming the person I always dreamed of. But those years I felt lost much of the time and I was looking for something that would fill that void. I would get into relationships that wouldn't even help the feeling. Obviously, I just didn't date someone because I felt lost or lonely. I cared about them a lot. It's just I didn't feel like I could connect and they'd understand what I'm going through. To be honest I am very happy that they didn't understand because to understand what I'm going through you would have to have gone through a hell of a lot of pain. The times I felt lonely and empty were the times I felt like I was dying. I'd wake up and be weaker even though I would train my butt off. I would try to gain weight by eating a lot but for some reason I'd lose weight. Everything I tried to do just didn't work out and those were the dark times for me. All I wanted was the comfort of knowing that it was okay if I didn't make it. But then I'd tell myself that it's not okay to give up and lose. I wasn't going to let a disease control the outcome. It's just hard to be strong every single day of your life when you are suffering so much. I'm incredibly strong but I'm not a robot at the same time either. For anyone who is going through something hard, it's okay to be down and it's okay to feel empty. You just can't quit, no matter what the task is.

I try every day to "win the day," as I call it. Did I do everything I could to bring myself closer to my goals? Did I work out? Did I try to stay strong and positive? If I did the majority of all these things, then I won the day. You're never going to win every day; it's just not how life is. When I would get down, I would try and find something to change my outlook, to change my perspective, regardless of the situation.

So, back to Bella. During those times I felt empty and lonely, that little five-pound animal made me feel so much better. Every time I was sick, she would come to me and bark to get on my bed so she could lie on my chest or lie next to me. If I was in a lot of pain, she would be there for me in a way I can't explain. She was like another family member—that's how I looked at it. She made me want to go outside and watch her run. Or take her on walks. She brought me joy during the worst time in my life. I was dying but when I was with her, I was happy. I never thought in a million years that a dog could have the power to do something like that. I'm telling you, every time I get upset that dog comes right to me. Now, I'm not saying my family doesn't do the same for me but when I get lonely or anxious, she makes me smile because of how cute she is. I'm telling you, Bella is so beautiful and she is so spoiled by me. That dog literally gets away with everything because of how much I love her.

The first year we had her, we were watching the Super Bowl. Now, my team is the Patriots because my dad is from Boston. My mom is from New York so I told myself, *I'll be a Yankees fan for her and I'll be a Patriots fan for Dad.* So back to what I was saying, it was half-time and the Patriots were winning and we had a party for it and I was very happy. I was feeling good, I had some friends over and it was overall a good night. Until Bella jumped off the couch and broke her leg. She was screaming so loud and I was so heartbroken. All I wanted to do was take her pain away and I couldn't. We took Bella to the vet where they took care of her and put her in a little pink cast.

The next week I had treatment and I was feeling awful. Now, mind you, Bella was in pain because she refused to take the pain meds. So I was feeling terrible and I was not happy because my dog was also in pain. She came to my bed again and barked to get up. She then settled down and slept on my chest because she knows that makes me feel better all the time. And that's my point, my dog knows when something is wrong. She knows when I'm in pain. She knows when I get anxious and nervous. And this time, even when she was in pain herself, Bella still came to me and helped me feel better.

Now, I'm not writing this to say everyone needs to go out and buy a dog. What I'm saying is: that dog helped to fill my heart. My family did the majority of it but Bella added to it and it was exactly what I needed. I'll be forever grateful for what my little girl did for me. In a weird way she made me want to fight even more. My family did the majority of it but she added to it. She helped me get out of bed when I was so sick. She helped me not feel lonely in my darkest times when I was dying. It was a beautiful thing. I think the more reasons you have to fight, the better chance you have to get what you want. Whether it's battling cancer, chasing a dream, or being a better person. The more reasons I had to fight, the better chance I had to achieve something. That's something I learned. It's hard to stay motivated every day. I get it, especially when you are so sick. But just think about the reasons why you need to fight. When you take the time to list every reason you have for fighting and not giving up, the better chance you have of getting out of bed and doing your thing.

Chapter 14

JOURNALING

"If you focus on what you left behind,
you will never see what lies ahead."
- Chef Gusteau, *Ratatouille*

THURSDAY

I woke up at 5:00 a.m., which is how I start each day. Every morning I wake up in pain, mainly because of the damage from the radiation and chemo. After I took my medicine, I immediately had a protein shake and drank a bottle of water.

Around 8:00 a.m., I shadow boxed with weighted gloves. I went 8 rounds. I like to do this every morning because it gets my body ready for the day. Gets my breathing better, muscles ready to go and all that.

Before boxing, I watched TV with my brother for a couple hours. I like watching TV in the morning, mostly shows and movies. Why? This just gets my mind off things so I can turn off my brain. Most nights I wake up in severe pain or I get woken up with a night terror. It's something I've unfortunately had to deal with because of everything that's happened to me.

I spent much of the afternoon speaking with my writing team about things I have to do for the book. They took my anxiety away and made me feel pretty excited about the whole thing. I like my book team. They encourage me, which gives me hope that my message will help others. So the pain and anxiety of everything gets channeled into writing, which helps me work things out somewhat.

After I was done writing, I did some cooking with my grandma. I really like cooking and find it fun and relaxing. My grandma has taught me so I'm pretty good in the kitchen. Tonight we had a lot of chicken and mashed potatoes. Mashed potatoes are my favorite. It's been that way since I was a kid.

Next up, another work out. I put in two hours of boxing with an elevation mask. The mask tests my breathing and it feels a million times harder to breathe. I'm not fighting in the ring currently. Boxing is definitely more than therapeutic; it keeps me in great shape. I love throwing my hands, so it's good all the way around.

Now I'm having a drink with my brother while watching TV. I'll be helping my grandparents get into bed soon. I take about 50 pills a day–vitamins, pain medicine because I have a lot of nerve and tissue damage, and anxiety medicine when I need it.

I only drink every so often but tonight's one of those nights. I'm getting closer to completing the book so I figured it was time to celebrate and a lot of work stuff is going well so what the hell you know. I just hope nothing happens while I sleep. It's really a 50/50 gamble, so we'll see.

FRIDAY

I woke up a bunch of times in the night because of pain and had a night terror. The reason these dreams are getting to me is because they are so real and I end up dying in them. Sometimes when I wake up, I can't even move for the first few minutes. Because of everything I've been through, my body is just reacting to the trauma of facing death. The weird thing is if I sleep with someone that I like (a girlfriend), I sleep like a baby. Very weird. I started my day doing 10 rounds of bag work. Took me about 40 minutes nonstop. After the workout, I showered, had a protein shake, and cooked some eggs and oatmeal. I then jumped back into writing some more. I will be doing this every day until I finish. The whole process is very exciting.

I finished writing at 4:00 p.m. Pretty tired, I mixed in some time for a nap or two. Between the workouts and the writing, I am often mentally and physically drained. I then helped with dinner. The menu consisted of kale, potatoes, chicken, and pasta. I usually eat dinner in my room while my family eats in the kitchen. I've been doing this ever since I got sick. I like to eat alone for some weird reason. After dinner, I lifted weights for another workout, showered, and went to bed.

I scheduled a call for Saturday with a family whose child has cancer. I prepared my notes for the call as I always do when I speak to the patient or the family. I've been doing this for years and I'm blessed that so many people have come to me for guidance and advice. I want to help them in any way I can. Helping people makes me the happiest and makes me feel like I'm changing lives in my own little way. The call was difficult because I know the pain that child and family were going through. I did my very best to give them hope because I believe hope is the most important thing to feel. Everything and anything is possible. I can't physically change their lives; all I can do is show them to the door but they have to be the ones to go through it. I know by the time the call was done that they felt hope. Later on I found out the child beat cancer! All I can do is share my story and my goal every time I talk with someone is to give hope, strength, and inspiration. If I don't do that, in my eyes I have failed. I give everything I have every time I make a call to someone who needs to talk, and when I do my job, it's the most amazing feeling.

After the call, the day ended as I took my medicine and put on a movie until I fell asleep.

SATURDAY

Last night was a good night. I slept nine hours without going to the bathroom, being in pain, or having a night terror. This sounds so weird but every time I put on an animated movie, like the kids' movie *Shrek* (love those movies), I seem to rest without night terrors. It's the most bizarre thing.

This week has been rough. My ex-girlfriend's mom passed away earlier this week so I've spent a lot of time trying to be there for her. Like every morning, I start the day by doing rounds of boxing. Did nine this morning. After that I took my meds of vitamins, anxiety meds, pain pills. Next, I made a protein shake and had an apple with eggs. Today I have two things I must do–work more on the book and talk to a family this afternoon. Every call I take I try to share something in my experience that can make them feel better. I've gotten quite good at this over the years. The most important thing is giving all these families hope. Hope, to me, gets you through a lot of things. Hope is believing good things are yet to come in whatever way that may be. At 2 o'clock I will be talking with this family. I am grateful that almost every time I talk, I share something from my journey that helps families feel a hell of a lot better. Maybe that's the positive of beating cancer so many times. I have something to offer and people really do listen and find some kind of encouragement, even if it is simply knowing they are not alone and the fight is worth the effort. Having beaten cancer five times, I'm getting pretty good at sharing how I fight the disease and hold on to hope. After every conversation with families, I feel better as well.

For the rest of the day, I helped my family around the house and helped cook dinner. I wanted to go to bed early because tomorrow is Mother's Day . I want to be rested and have a strong day for her.

SUNDAY

So today I woke up really early to make some Mother's Day cards. After making the cards, I went to the florist. My mom and grandmother love roses and I brought home two dozen. We had a nice celebration when I returned. This time together was good. They do so much for me. Seems crazy that we only allocate one day a year as Mother's Day.

Well, the routine continues. Being committed to getting stronger through my fitness routine means sticking to it even on Mother's Day. So breakfast is a protein shake and eggs with turkey bacon. Next I go to the garage and work out where I did 10 four-plus minutes rounds. My punches are getting faster and heavier, which I'm pretty excited about. While I was hitting the bag, I wore my elevation mask on the highest level. Once I finished 10 rounds nonstop, I decided to lift weights. To time my rounds, I use my YouTube app and play songs. The songs range from 4 minutes to 4 minutes and 50 seconds. This is how I break down 40 minutes of nonstop boxing, 10 four-minute songs. It is a challenge but for me, the fight is as much mental as physical, and strengthening my mind helps fight the battle as well.

After I worked out, I showered and cleaned up because the rest of the day consisted of the family spoiling my mom and Grandma. We did the cooking, drove them anywhere they wanted to go, watched some movies with them and more. It was truly "their day." Dad and I fired up the grill to barbeque and after we were done eating, we showered Mom and Grandma with presents. Today was a busy day. And once the celebrating was over, I hung out with my brother, then went to bed early because I have to leave in the morning for my next round of treatment. We leave the house at 6:30 a.m. to be there by 7:00 a.m. for the blood work. Once the results come in, I typically wait 30 minutes to an hour before chemotherapy is administered.

MONDAY

Today I woke up at 4:45 a.m. because I like to have some time to myself before we leave at 6:30. I did 8 rounds of shadow boxing with weighted gloves, then had a shake and took my medicine. With the time left, I started watching a show with my brother before he started work. We watch reality TV. It's kind of funny and very entertaining. The little things can be a real escape and a small about of "time off" is good for my frame of mind.

At 6:30 I got in the car and we arrived at the hospital at 7:00. By 7:15 they took my blood and did my vitals.

Two and a half months ago I weighed 242 pounds and my resting heart rate was 127. I now weigh 221 and my resting heart rate is 79. This means my heart is healthier and stronger. After the pneumonia I promised myself I would breathe well and be in crazy shape. For two years I was doing strongman workouts. I gained over 75 pounds and was the size of a refrigerator and I felt like one. I'm still big but I look much more toned and I'm more healthy for sure.

While I was getting chemo, I had a telehealth with my oncologist. She was thrilled with everything and said I was doing absolutely amazing with my blood counts. My cardio is just boxing because it helps me deal with my anxiety and is crazy good for you. Because of it I'm in crazy shape. After chemo I got home and had breakfast, which was eggs and oatmeal. Then I did 12 rounds on the heavy bag without stopping or sitting down, then lifted weights for almost 40 minutes.

I showered and took a nap because I was feeling tired. Once I woke up from my nap I spoke to a family and tried giving them hope about their son who has leukemia. I think I did a great job because at the beginning of the call they were crying and at the end of it they sounded strong and were laughing so that made me feel good.

Most days I have chemo, I take it easy but I always train. It's very hard to do it and that's exactly why I don't take a day off. I stay strong every day and am constantly trying to accomplish new things and be a better me. I try to be smarter, stronger, and do so many different things every day. I never waste a day, that's for sure. None are promised to us and I am someone who knows this truth for certain.

It was a good day. This evening, I had steak and potatoes for dinner. I then took my meds and went to bed at 7:00 pm. In the night I woke up with a bad night terror and woke up three times in crazy pain. All I could do was take my medicine and pray. Praying gives me strength and makes my anxiety go down. I slept in that morning. The days I have chemo I sleep a lot because I do so much by getting up early, working out, getting to the hospital, not to mention the toll the chemo takes.

TUESDAY

The day after chemo is always the hardest on me but nothing changes. I felt bad because I woke up screaming in the craziest amount of pain. Luckily nobody woke up, but once the pain subsided, which was about 3:30 a.m., I couldn't fall back to sleep so I watched some movies. At 5:00 a.m. I did some cardio. I did 10 rounds on the heavy bag using my music mix to help me get about 40 minutes of workout. I sat down for maybe 10 seconds once because my right leg, which is the weakest, had spasms. My right leg is weakest because during my journey with cancer I had a 13-cm (the size of an orange) mass in my hip. The radiation, while taking it away, caused a lot of nerve damage and left me with a lot of scar tissue. I also was injured during strongman training. While doing the log clean and press, I fell with the log right on my knee. So, with all those things I have a slight limp so it makes boxing difficult. I was really cranking that bag. I was hitting it so hard and was doing 10 straight rounds on the highest level with the elevation mask.

Once I was done, I showered and made myself breakfast consisting of a protein shake, eggs, and oatmeal. While eating, I answered emails and messages from people asking for my advice on their battle with cancer. Much of the other work was responding to work-related emails.

Because the day after chemo the pain is at its worst, I get very nauseated but to keep going, I had to learn to deal with it and move on. Later in the day my grandmother and I shopped for my youngest brother's birthday presents. His birthday is next week. Yes we are a card and gift-giving family. It's always been that way.

I laid low and rested after shopping because I had done my training and everything else my day called for. At dinner I wasn't really hungry so I had a bowl of cereal. I love cinnamon cereal. It's my go-to when nothing else sounds good.

I ended up watching TV with my brother and passed out. Not much of a crazy day but that's what I did. Slept well till about 2:00 a.m., then had a terrible night terror during which I woke up in a complete sweat. Once I fell back to sleep, the pain woke me up again and this was bad, I couldn't walk till the medicine kicked in. I push myself harder and harder every day so it's not surprising that my body is reacting this violently. I want to be in the best physical shape possible so when the day comes when it looks like it's the end for me, I'm as strong as I can be. My body and mind are focused on prepping for the worst, while hoping for the best. I promised myself after my fourth bout with pneumonia that I would never have such a hard time breathing again. So, I choose to do crazy amounts of cardio every day and I'm breathing better than I did when I was in my best boxing condition. Every time I work out now, I use that elevation mask and it really has taken my lungs to the next level of fitness.

WEDNESDAY

I was up all night and it was pretty rough. I was in pain the entire night. I didn't have a night terror, thankfully, but I kept waking up in extreme pain. The pain meds weren't helping so I was either tossing and turning or I was walking around and stretching. My hip felt like someone swung a bat at it and made full contact. My spine felt like I was getting poked with needles from top to bottom. These nights don't happen as often but I think because of how hard I train it has something to do with it. Last year when I had pneumonia, I promised myself I will have the strongest lungs and be in the best shape possible while still being very strong. Every time I work out my grandparents watch me and they always say how great I did but are so confused as to why I push myself the way I do. Every time I train, I train as if my life is on the line and I think of the moments where I thought I was going to die and it pushes me harder and harder. I think exercising and pushing myself while battling cancer is so important. It keeps my body strong so when I go to battle I have my best shot. I stress this with everyone with health issues. When you do well with your self-training, you get this sense of pride because you know you are working hard to keep your body strong.

At 5:00 a.m., I started my morning rounds of shadow boxing with weighted gloves. I did about 10 or 12 rounds nonstop and each round was accompanied by YouTube songs. That four to five-minute duration for each song gives me a mental marker and push, knowing 10 to 12 rounds requires I just get through two to three songs. I finished around 6:15 a.m., drenched in sweat and in heavy pain. But I remembered last year when I had pneumonia. I remembered how on the first day I got home from the hospital, I couldn't get up a half of a flight of stairs. And I thought to myself, Dang, it wasn't that long ago that I was able to do all those rounds nonstop with an elevation mask at the hardest level. Throwing thousands and thousands of punches with weighted gloves is hard but it felt great. After I was done, I went into the shower and said to myself, My God, I'm strong. I went from almost dead to feeling this energized and fit. This feeling is something that fuels my drive, especially when I know I am facing another round of chemo. If the training doesn't kill me, the cancer doesn't have a fighting chance.

After my shower I made breakfast for my grandparents and me consisting of eggs, toast, hash browns, kale, and oatmeal. Once I was done, I proceeded to focus on writing the book until lunch time. Because I didn't sleep at all last night and I was still in pain, I decided to put heating pads on the areas that hurt and take time to rest. It was time for my brother's work break so we hung out and watched TV. After resting for a bit, I felt strong enough and highly motivated to get coffee with this girl I like named Clair. She is very beautiful, a sweet girl, and I had some fun writing to her as a way to get to know each other.

When I returned home, it was workout time again. I do all these rounds in the morning mainly to get my lungs going and I like to start each day breaking a sweat. Not a normal sweat but the kind of drenching that feels like diving into a pool. This workout was another 1,000 punches thrown with weighted gloves and of course my elevation mask at the top level. Around 4 o'clock that afternoon, I started my powerlifting program which took me about 45 minutes to complete with the elevation mask for maximum breathing impact.

After the powerlifting, I hit the bag with the weighted gloves for 7 rounds (30 minutes). I then went inside, showered, and ate dinner. My grandma and I cooked a vegetable and steak dinner earlier in the day, so the food was ready. After eating, I had another phone call, this time with a family whose daughter has leukemia. I tried to give the family hope and strength and help them believe God has a plan for them that they will get through. The daughter, Lilly, was scared as she was starting chemo soon. I told her not to be scared and that chemo gives you superpowers. And she got all excited and that made the parents feel better because the daughter wasn't sad. I then asked the parents if Lilly has something she has dreamed of doing but not yet accomplished. They said she wants to go horseback riding. I told them I know someone who is a professional horse rider and that I would make the call tomorrow to see if we can get a horseback riding day scheduled. I told the parents my Foundation would help pay for the riding experience. After that call I went to bed because I didn't sleep much last night and wanted to get some rest.

THURSDAY

In the middle of the night I woke up in a lot of pain again. I really do believe the training is increasing my pain. I'm not injuring muscles or overworking things. I have a lot of nerve damage and scar tissue. At night the pain seems to get more intense. It's weird that when the weather changes for the worse, the pain gets more intense. Because I'm sleeping better, I'm not taking any medicine, so when I do wake up, it's with the feeling of just having had the crap kicked out of me. Sometimes I wake up cursing because I am sleeping well and then, BAM, my body hurts everywhere. I then take some pain medicine and within a half hour the pain eases. I will be doing physical therapy soon. I just want to get my Covid vaccine shots first before I go into a physical therapy treatment facility.

The last week's sleeping patterns have been rough for me. Pain in the middle of the night combined with night terrors are really tough for me. It just happens. I know the training adds to it, but the training makes me feel better emotionally and physically. I would love to compete in future boxing matches or a strongman competition. Training for these events is what keeps me working out so much. Even if I don't compete, the boxing and breathing work gets and keeps me in such amazing shape. If I have to suck it up to make sure I'm healthy, then so be it. It's part of both my physical and mental strength preparation and building. So, today I woke up around 3:00 a.m. with the pain and couldn't fall back to sleep. So, at 5:30 a.m., I went to the garage and got the bag for 10 rounds which took me about 40-45 minutes nonstop with the elevation mask on the highest level with weighted gloves. Once I finish and go inside, I take off my mask and sit on the couch and my breathing feels amazing. My mom is working out as well, doing her 12 miles on the bike then 2 miles on the treadmill. She likes to be the first one in the shower so I wait for her to get done then jump in and take mine.

Next I have my protein shake while I make breakfast for my grandparents and me. Today it's eggs, turkey bacon, oatmeal, and coffee for the three of us. After breakfast I wrote a few hours. I'm trying to get the book done as fast as possible. I feel a sense of urgency to get the message out to share with the world. I have a lot going with the book, career, and opportunities to share my story and help people, which makes me happy, but things will really get moving in full gear when the book comes out. This is an important project for me, so it keeps me thinking and working hard to get it done. I took my break at around 11:00 a.m. which turned into a short nap because getting up at 3:00 a.m. takes a toll. After the nap I had two calls with two families. One family is facing cancer with a child and the other the wife is in her battle. I am grateful for the opportunity to speak with families. Being part of a support system for others gives me energy and a sense of giving back. Because the training continues to build my strength and confidence (despite the pain), I will get a powerlifting session in tonight but I am giving the punching bag a rest this evening.

I made myself some lunch today as well, which was a steak and asparagus. I'm trying to take it easy and spend time with my brother. His birthday is next week and he will be away from home for a month when it's my birthday, so I want to spend as much time as possible with him. Time is very valuable and important to me. Spending it with my family is important and I want as much of it as possible with them. This evening I help my grandfather cook dinner around 5:00 p.m. I do this almost every night and that's it for my day. Good night!

I am still in pain almost every day, but the medicine really does help, thankfully. It may sound morbid but I'd rather be in pain from training than stop training and possibly be dead. I'm always pushing to be better and stronger every day. I have been this way since I was diagnosed all those years ago.

JOURNAL
LAST 30 DAYS

I guess what I'll start with is the first day of every month. I have chemotherapy. I wake up at 5:00 a.m. even though I leave at 6:30 because I like to have some time to myself before I to go into chemo. I calm my mind, visualize the process, focus on my mindset. It's like going into battle. I need my mindset on MY team. The chemo alone is hard enough. Getting my mindset to accept the day will be a team effort and when the physical is taking a hit, the mental (mindset) needs to step up. This month I did five rounds of five-minute treatment. Mental and physical played as a team. After each chemo round I pushed to do my workouts (thanks, mindset) then head inside from my garage gym and shower. The feeling and the look of my body responding to the workouts gives me more confidence and drive to keep working and keep fighting. It's crazy but I want the hospital staff and caregivers to see that I am working as hard as they are and that the battle goes on well after they administer my treatment. Chemo is only part of the fight. I guess it's a combination of things which must go into a holistic battle. How can I expect the best results if I don't commit fully to the war and battle every day to the best of my ability? The caregivers all know me at the hospital. I know they care about me, so when they see that I am putting in the work physically outside of my treatments, I know it makes them feel good. Plus, here is the real question I ask myself often and the one that pushes me. How can I speak with families who are facing the same battle that I am and NOT bring every ounce of my mind, body, and spirit to my fight to be the example of what I am speaking to them?

When I had pneumonia last year, I had put in a ton of work with weightlifting. I was 240 pounds, not fat but very strong. I was doing strongman training after we won the fight of my brain cancer diagnosis. I set a personal goal to compete in the strongman program and the work required to get ready built muscle, which made me bigger and as strong as I had ever been. After I beat brain cancer, I weighed 147 pounds. So, I gained a lot of muscle. I received a real scare when during that training my resting heart rate was sitting at 127bpm. Not good.

I promised myself after my fourth battle with pneumonia, I would never struggle with breathing like that again. I would work to get into the best overall shape possible. This meant cardio fitness as well. So, I started boxing and my resting heart rate went from 127 bpm to 77 bpm in six months. The high resting heart rate resulted from the body building AND all the treatments I endured. So the switch to add all the cardio (boxing and breathing apparatus) was for safety and to get more holistically healthy. I'm still big but I'm leaner with muscles that are more defined and cut. Given the spike in heart rate, every time I go into the hospital for treatment, I am more nervous about my heart rate than anything. I've lost 20 pounds but the only reason why I didn't lose more is because I gained more muscle from boxing and powerlifting. Walking and moving is now so much easier, which gives me more confidence and a more positive mindset.

My next treatment, I get called in at 8:00 a.m. They usually have to try four or five times to get the IV set in me because my veins are shot from all the chemo. I didn't have a port installed when I had transplants. Why? I knew if a port was installed I would not be able to box. I couldn't risk getting punched in the port. Plus, I didn't want something popping out of my chest. I know this might sound vain, but that's how I felt. I'm sure one day I'll need it but for now we passed on the port and deal with finding a good vein each time. I guess you can say that I traded vain for vein. My treatment takes 40 minutes. I then go home, talk to my doctor, and I rest. I have to rest more on the days of chemo but later in the afternoon I train for an hour or so. The motivation to work out so much through the treatment is because I conduct calls with families and individuals in the evenings. We speak about their child or family member with cancer, or I talk directly to the person going through the cancer treatment. I like to do this because I'm doing my part in making a difference. The physical training helps in two ways. First, it gives me the energy and mindset that if I can push myself through the workouts, that the disease can't beat me. Second, I am more energized to encourage the patients and families to do THEIR FIGHT. I let them know that they and their bodies can do more than they might think. This helps me and I believe helps those I speak with.

After the first day of chemo, I do all the normal life stuff including the workouts daily. I also love cooking. It is very relaxing for me and it allows me to spend time with my grandmother every day. The more cooking I do, the better I am getting at it. Another challenge for me to tackle.

The past month I have committed much of my time for calls with the partnerships I have as part of my Foundation. I have a manager who sets these appointments for me. More is coming around these partnerships and the Foundation this year which I'm very happy about.

As far as my social life, I am dating, which gets me out of the house a couple times a month. I am having a good time. While I don't have a serious relationship, dating does bring back a sense of normalcy to life. While I haven't found the right one yet, I'm sure it'll happen.

Planning and goals are also important as part of my routine. At the first of each month while at chemotherapy, I write in the notes app on my phone the things I plan to accomplish. Some of those things are how much writing I will do this month, my fitness goals of getting more and more in shape every month and to do everything I can to grow stronger and to feel healthier. I aim to help someone at least each week, by being on a call giving some guidance to families on what to do about their child being sick (I do this very often) or even something as simple as helping my grandparents drive to New York and visit the gravesite of my uncle who recently passed away. I'm always trying to make a difference in the lives of others and my whole career is now focused on making a difference. I mean, a real difference. I know if I can do that, then everything I've been through will have been a blessing. It's really the main thing that keeps me fighting. Otherwise, what would this all be worth? My experiences have given me the opportunity to face a huge set of challenges and to become stronger through them. Now I can share my experiences about developing both mental and physical toughness. This is the big stuff. Of course we always have the conversations about what to expect day to day during treatment, but the big message is to get in there and fight with everything you have. The more you fight the more others will fight with you. One of the toughest lessons for me was realizing that I had to grow up pretty fast. When you start fighting at 19, you really do grow up pretty fast. The little things that used to bother me are gone. What seemed critical before cancer melts away, and the meaning of life comes into focus fast and pretty clearly.

When you first look at me, you'd never know I was sick. I look like an athlete and most importantly I look very healthy. But the reality is there are lots of things I deal with on a daily basis which are tough for me. I'm in pain all the time and I'm lucky that I have a great pain management doctor and the medicine I get really does help a lot, but I wake up every morning in so much pain. Some nights I wake up screaming because of the night terrors I have due to PTSD. When I work out, I'm always in so much pain from all the nerve damage from all the radiation treatments my body has endured.

I'm starting physical therapy soon, but I wanted to start once I got my Covid shot and hopefully the physical therapy will be able to make my body feel less destroyed and more connected and engaged. One example of a current limitation that I want to eliminate is that I can't run. While I was doing strongman, I was overhead pressing a log and it fell right on my knee. I don't want to have surgery, so we are going to try physical therapy. After some PT treatment, I'll find out if surgery will be required. I can't move as well boxing right now, but the more I move in the ring, the stronger my knee is becoming. It's hard to move around and when I throw punches, the pain is intense. I've worked hard to develop and maintain my strength. However what I believe has strengthened the most is my mindset. I have had to fight every excuse in the book which would have made it so easy to quit in every battle. My commitment to myself is to get and stay healthy. I strive to be the best I can be no matter how much I suffer.

My struggle is real, and I try to share with families that they have to embrace all emotions. The mindset swings happen. Out of nowhere I can be laughing or just watching TV and then, all of a sudden, I have a panic attack. This is something that makes me nervous when I go out and socialize because folks might not understand and I don't want them to be uncomfortable. I don't want an awkward situation but, such is life. I know I shouldn't be embarrassed about the emotional swings but they happen. I have some medicine that helps. In some cases I just think of something that gets my mind off the situation for a minute. Often it's a feeling or anger versus panic. Not sure why but I have to do whatever it takes. There is no manual to follow for dealing with the emotional aspect. In all of life we have to find ways to cope and overcome.

I love my life. I really do. I thank God every day for giving me the opportunity to do the things I do and to be alive after everything I've been through. My life isn't perfect. I have things I deal with on a daily basis, but I'd rather have all those things happen and be alive then to not be alive at all. My father said something to me that I never forgot. Years ago when I was struggling with the pain, he said, "You have to learn to be comfortable with being uncomfortable." I think of that every day while I'm in pain or I'm having a panic attack. I don't have a perfect life but I can promise you that I will get what I've always wanted, which is for my story to make a worldwide difference because I know it will help people. So, in my down time I try to figure out how to do it. I have a great team and we are on our way to getting there.

Now other things that get me through the challenges are the times I watch movies with my brothers. I love doing that because 1) I love movies and 2) I love spending time with my brothers. I like to just hang out with them when they aren't working because we are so close. But I do have times when I'm alone, which is a good amount of time, and I tend to get depressed. But I don't feel sorry for myself. I'm just sick of being in pain all the time and every time I leave my house, I have to have a medicine bag with me. It frustrates me. When I go on dates or hang out with my friends, I'm always nervous I'm going to have a panic attack. But these are things I have to deal with. There were a handful of times I thought I was going to die and I'm blessed God gave me strength to keep pushing and keep fighting along with giving me a family that never quit on me. Without those things I wouldn't here.

The people who are reading this don't feel amazing all the time. I have my problems just like each and every one of you. But what I do is I never quit. It's tempting to not go out on a date because I'm afraid I might have a panic attack, or because my limp might make me look weird. But I choose to go out and socialize anyway. I always do things I want to do and I don't let my insecurities or fear stop me from living because living is the most important thing. My pain will get better, my PTSD will get better. I just hold on and keep moving forward and if you are reading this, here is my advice to you: Do the things that you are afraid of; take chances; do something you never thought you could do. Always fight and never give up because if you quit, the things you are afraid of will keep you from creating the best memories of your life. Everything and anything is possible. I think about these things every day. I choose to accomplish anything I want to and I fight for it because I believe I can do anything, Yes, sometimes I doubt myself but once I get myself together, I take a few deep breaths and figure out how to pursue what I want.

I'm not perfect by any means. But what I do is fight and when I'm down I get back up. So, when I have my moments of depression, experience physical pain, or have a panic attack, I tell myself all these things will pass. The pain and anxiety will pass after I take my prescribed medicine.

I'm alone a lot and my brain is always in motion. I'm always thinking and I try to be as productive as possible. When I'm alone I like to spend time with my dog, Bella. I love her so much for what she did for me while I was pushing to fight brain cancer. I take her on walks and we love being outside together. And when I'm not feeling well because of the chemo or for any other reason, I like to spend time with my Bella. Weekends are my favorite part of the week because my family isn't working and I get to spend a lot of time with them. I love my family more than anything and something as simple as sitting on the porch talking with my mom or dad or my grandparents makes me happy. We play corn hole or whatever games we have. I'm just happy that I'm getting closer and closer to my dreams and most importantly, I'm living. Regardless of how many problems I have and even though I'll have to do chemo for the rest of my life, I'll still make sure to be happy and do what I love.

Most days are similar but, to be honest, even though I'm doing better than ever I still get depressed sometimes. There's no explanation or reason why but sometimes I'll be sitting there and just get sad. Usually when that happens, I try to do something to get my mind off of things. For example, I'll play with my dogs and take them for a walk. I'll watch a movie that makes me laugh. Or I will spend time with friends doing fun things like rock climbing, ax throwing, or bowling. A lot of times though when I get depressed, I work out. I know I say I do it a lot but it really does make me feel better. Whether it's powerlifting or boxing, I always feel better after working out.

The big problem is when I'm feeling down or depressed, there's a high chance I'll have a panic attack. I love my life, I really do. I got through the toughest things anyone can go through but I'm definitely not fully recovered emotionally and physically.

I get treatment once every month. I most often get depressed during the week I have chemo. Just being reminded of all the pain and suffering I go through is tough to deal with. And when I'm in the hospital I feel bad because there are so many people that are really sick and are in wheelchairs. Then I remember when I myself was in a wheelchair and I feel proud for having gotten myself out of it. But then I feel bad that I put my family through this. This battle wasn't just affecting me, it affected everyone who cares for me. I just want people to know it's okay to get down on yourself or feel depressed. I deal with it all the time. But I do my very best to pull myself up out of depression by doing those things that help. I think of those activities as my tools for changing my mindset and making it more positive. Everyone's different and you can find your own tools–that is, find those things that help you feel more positive and that bring you joy when you're down.

I'm so blessed that God has given me the strength to fight the way I do. He has helped me to turn the difficulties in my life into something good–which is helping people. I'm not perfect by any means but these are the things I deal with regularly as I go through the routine of monthly chemo. It seems the farther I get away from the chemo, the less depressed or down I feel. For example, after the first week of the chemo I feel better mentally. And also, physically.

Now, this treatment is the best I've ever been on. It keeps my cancer away and it has minimal side effects. I feel tired for the first week or two and I get very itchy but it goes away. I try not to dwell on these negatives. I learned to do the things I love the most in order to fight through the negative thoughts and feelings. Every time I get down, I think to myself, I got through it and I did it. And I remind myself that the situation I'm in right now is a million times better than what it was. And I'm sure a lot of people can relate to that in the sense that they've been through something bad and they realized they got through it and they are still here. Now I know I've said it before but every month I feel this way and I know it'll only get better from here. Dealing with the fact I'm going to need treatment for the rest of my life was difficult to hear but as long as I'm doing what I love and I'm happy, then that's all that matters.

Every day, I try to be as productive as possible, especially the week of treatment. When I get all these things done–whether it's doing something for work, or training, helping someone on the phone, or even just helping around the house–I take it as a win. Because the treatment leaves me tired and in pain, I have every excuse to lie in bed. Instead, I choose to push myself and do even more because I realize neither the illness nor the treatment has killed me, and that makes me feel good.

Chapter 15

REACTION TO BEING DIAGNOSED AND WHERE I STAND NOW

"Start by doing what's necessary; then do what's possible; and suddenly you are doing the impossible."
-Francis of Assisi

When I was diagnosed, it was not as bad as some people might think. Before the cancer diagnosis, something else happened that I thought of as the most devastating thing I could experience. Most of my life had been committed to the sport I loved, hockey. I loved the game and worked tirelessly to become the best I could be. This work had me focused on trying to earn a college scholarship, which was my dream. And I did earn that scholarship. Then, everything changed when I was hit by a car and broke my leg. My hockey career was over. BAM! My dream was shattered.

After the car accident, I lost all that I had worked for up to that moment. Still, I told myself I had to make something of my life. I took a pre-law class and my teacher inspired me to pursue a law degree. I saw this as a way to help others. My teacher spoke eighteen languages and had worked with President Obama. For the first time in my life I studied as hard as I could. I took the energy which had been invested in hockey and now funneled it into studying. The result from my efforts got me straight A's and an acceptance letter to Fordham University. I wasn't just proud of myself for acceptance to Fordham. My pride grew because I knew that no teacher would have ever believed I would be accepted there. Getting in was hard work but my first semester of my sophomore year was a true nightmare. I had vertigo almost the entire semester and had crazy night sweats virtually every night. My body also started to itch uncontrollably. The itching was unbearable. There were so many signs that things weren't going my way. I was getting knocked down and when I got back up, I was knocked down again.

I lost 40 pounds that semester and I knew something wasn't right with my body but I never thought it would be cancer. After seeing twelve doctors they finally made the correct diagnosis. Yes indeed, it was cancer.

What was so bizarre was that before the diagnosis, I was taking a class in communications. My only project for the class was to give a presentation on a particular topic. The topic that I chose was cancer. Doing research on a topic can be rather emotionless if it is not of real interest to or of great impact on the student. But when I got the call saying I was diagnosed with a massive tumor in my chest, my research became personal. All the research I had done on cancer made me realize how serious my diagnosis was. I realized this was going to be another challenge for me to face and tackle.

I wasn't really scared. I did however begin feeling nervous and anxious in the waiting room before they called me in for my first chemo. I was awake all night looking for a message, a person, a quote—anything really—to inspire me. I wanted to know I wasn't going to be sick and in bed all day throwing up.

What do people do to stay strong, positive, and focused on conquering this awful condition? How do they get through this? I wanted stories of folks that fought and beat it. I was determined to be a victor just as I had been when life threw me challenges before. I had risen to the top in my hockey journey, done the work, faced the obstacles, and earned top accolades. I decided that was how I was going to attack cancer. Same mindset, different battle. Unfortunately, I couldn't really find much about people doing things like pursuing a sport, a workout program, something strenuous physically while going through cancer treatment. This was always my way of dealing with challenges. I would work harder, put in more time, more repetitions, more hours on the ice.

Knowing that with cancer I would be in a lot of pain and sick and potentially not able to do anything to fight it scared me the most. For the first time in my life I wasn't going to be an athlete, and I didn't know any way other than sports to meet my challenges and to face my demons. This is what scared me the most. As you know, my cancer came back a second time. It was at this point that I told myself I WILL be an athlete. I will do something that I am used to and that pushes me to be my best and to be something that I'm proud of. I couldn't skate, but what I did find was boxing. When I put on the gloves and either hit the bag or climbed in the ring, I could go on for hours and hours. I didn't break down or wear down like those around me thought I would. My energy was so focused and channeled into throwing punches. This was my way of hitting back and beating back at life, which I felt kept screwing me over. This was my way of saying NOT TODAY CANCER. The more punches I threw without collapsing the stronger my resolve became to stay in both the boxing ring and in the fight to beat the diagnosis that kept coming at me.

This work, my belief in myself, and the support of so many around me has gotten my cancer under control. If I have any cancer, it's a very small amount. Yes, I deal with it through regular treatment and all the routines required. But with all we are committed to doing (fighting the good fight) it won't affect me. We have been sustaining the fight and I am excited because we have been winning.

The way my doctor explains my treatment is that my cancer will fluctuate. For example, last year they found two dangerous spots in my body. One was in my quadriceps; that is, in my thigh. If the spot grew larger, I would be unable to walk. The second area was high risk as well and showed up in my spine. In these cases, I had to undergo radiation as a step to prevent the cancer from getting worse. When someone receives radiation, they make a mold for use when on the radiation table. You have to strip down to just your underwear and they make tattoos (a dot) on your body so they know the exact point for the radiation to penetrate each time. They take a needle and inject black ink on the exact area. The point of this is when you are on the machine they know where to do the radiation. I have over 50+ dots on my body. These dots are small but the process is very uncomfortable because you are practically naked in front of a dozen strangers. This is another reason I work out so hard. Gotta look good for the caregivers, right?

About a month after the initial markings and scans, my radiologist, who is the best, ordered another scan of the original spots to see if there had been any changes in size. I found out before Christmas last year the area of cancer was gone so I didn't need the radiation. Little wins are really something to get excited about. I will continue to get brain scans as well every six months. These scans will continue until I am cancer free for five to six years. And because this last scan was so good, I won't get my next scan for another six to maybe nine months.

Winning these battles gives me greater commitment to keep fighting the war. Little wins also remove some of the stress of the unknown. NOT TODAY CANCER! Even though the radiation is working for me and I am grateful for its effect, it has caused permanent damage and creates pain in my hip and back almost every day. When I'm training, the pain is always there and at times unbearable, but I just suck it up and get the workouts done because they are not only something I love but they are keeping me strong and healthy. I never get nervous about whether the radiation works or not because it always has. It's just that the damage it causes is impactful and I know it has lasting impact. While I don't know the extent, I do know there are adverse side effects. I will be getting radiation every day for two weeks and I think about the impact every day. I have to believe that killing the cancer will occur before the side effects get me. Again, the workouts, the physical and mental training I do works with the whole program. The chemotherapy and radiation attack the cancer, I work out and attack the punching bag. Together we are FIGHTING the cancer. I'm saying all this because it's something I think about every day. Every time I feel a pinch or a discomfort, I always question if it's cancer and that makes me anxious. So, imagine wondering every time you feel a pinch or a chest pain whether you have cancer. I deal with this every day. But I remain confident because I'm getting stronger, fitter, healthier every day as well. Cancer isn't the end. For me it has become my daily quest to get stronger, live better, help more people, strengthen my resolve, challenge my mental strength. We only grow if we are stretching ourselves. If for some reason my situation changes, I will not stop working or training. That is NOT an option. I will fight it till I win but most importantly no matter how bad it is or how scared I am that something will be taken from me, I tell myself I can and will do this no matter what. And I will keep telling myself that and working until the anxiety goes away.

When you've been battling for so long, you can't help but to think about it and I'm sure there are people out there who can understand that. I choose to be positive. I had a ring made when I was 21 years old. When I'm nervous about my cancer I take the ring off and read the word inscribed on the inside. The word is FEARLESS. And that's something I've strived to be ever since I got this ring. Anytime in my life that something scares me, even if it's not cancer, I take the ring off and read it till the fear goes away and that's something that helps me. Now I know I'm getting a little off topic but these are the things I deal with even though we see the cancer fading and especially when I don't have cancer anymore, I'm sure "FEARLESS" will remain my word. Is there really any other way to face life and beat down any obstacle?

Chapter 16

WHAT'S GOING ON WITH MY BODY

"Getting Comfortable With Being Uncomfortable"

The August before I was diagnosed with cancer, I started having a strong itching sensation in my feet. By September, I felt the itch from head to toe. No matter how I cleaned my body or whatever I put in it, the itch was insatiable and unrelenting. While in my college classes, I sat in the back of the classroom, took off my boots, and scratched myself with a pen. This was in addition to my feeling of vertigo and blurred eyesight. I had experienced poison ivy before and the itch I had was much worse. What seemed crazy is there were no rashes on my skin. Every time I showered, I destroyed my entire body scratching it to the point where I broke my skin and bled. I went to over a dozen doctors that fall and no one could diagnose the cause or condition. Two doctors said the itch was in my head. Every second of every day I was scratching some part of my body. It was driving me crazy and as the days went by the itch was so severe, I would scratch myself with anything sharp. I had cuts from head to toe and my skin felt like it was on fire. Even without clothes the itch was relentless. Imagine being in an intimate situation with a girlfriend or spouse and you can't help but be incessantly scratching yourself. Not my idea of being in the moment. I constantly thought to myself, "Why won't this stop?" My feet were the worst. I was in so much pain and felt like I was losing my mind. Finally, in December my mom took me to my old dermatologist who treated me for acne during high school. The doctor wanted me to do lighting treatments. I'll never forget her face when she saw what my body looked like covered in bruises, cuts, and scabs from head to toe. I told her during the visit that the itch gets way worse after a shower. Her face lit up and she knew exactly what to do. She ordered a chest X-ray. We got an appointment at the hospital that day and a couple hours later I was diagnosed with cancer.

The itching went away after my first chemotherapy treatment. Chemo started in the new year. My diagnosis came just three days before Christmas. I remember opening up my presents and saying, "Thank you, Mom and Dad, for the clothing, but I can't wear any of the items because they will aggravate the itching." My saying this and the fact that I had cancer broke their hearts. I still feel bad about that day but at that moment I wasn't thinking straight. Having vertigo for months, itching myself every five seconds, not seeing straight, commuting to school, and trying to learn how to study when I couldn't see made being a thoughtful son rather difficult at the moment.

The day after my first chemotherapy treatment, the itch went away completely. Yes, I was so sick, but I was so happy for the itch to go away. You learn things after the first couple years with cancer. If the itching starts up again, I know my cancer is getting worse. Once it starts, I know I'm not in good shape. But from of all the treatments I've had over the past 12 years, there are also other causes of having an itching sensation. This time it is bearable and not at all like what it was. I was tortured every second of every day. Now, it is more under control.

I had an apartment at school with my brother and that semester with the itch I remember sometimes I'd wake up bleeding because I had scratched myself in my sleep. One time my ex-girlfriend got blood on her and I felt really bad about that. But again, none of this is my fault. To this day, I can still get pretty itchy. But thank God for a good moisturizer which takes the itching away for a while. There was so much going on in all those months before I was diagnosed. It took over a dozen doctors to figure out what was wrong with me. The worst part about it was being told it was in my head. Well, thank God for the dermatologist who understood the symptoms of the itching getting worse after a shower.

I was supposed to be at a different university playing hockey. But the dream of hockey was gone and I was at Fordham, and I kept telling myself, "I'm at a great school and I'm going to make something of myself." I was just in a lot of physical and mental pain during that semester when everything started. Those four months were a lot to deal with, but I just tried getting through it day by day. A lot was going on but I just tried to deal with everything and take it in stride like I believed anyone else would. I never thought in a million years would it be cancer but hey, it is what it is, you know? During those four months, I had to learn how to study when I couldn't really see and let me tell you that was hard. No audio books or tutors to read aloud for me. I also had chest pains every so often. The pain was very strong and the place I got them was where my cancer was growing. Vertigo, itch, and the stress from school were the toughest things. I tried to study and work out. I didn't party because I already had blurry vision. I was also getting more and more tired.

Now, 12 years later, I'm doing well and am proud of myself. I'm so strong and my breathing/cardio is so good. One downside is the chemotherapy and radiation treatments. They take a toll and are like going through a hockey career of constant body checks into the boards. I have scar tissue damage as well as nerve damage. So without my pain medication, I would suffer pretty badly. I also have PTSD from all the things I went through, and have panic attacks that very often leave me thinking I might die. The panic attacks are real and often very present in my life. But one thing I have learned about myself is that I know how to fight and am very willing to fight. I know how to fight back and do a hell of a job doing it. Even though my anxiety and pain are still present in my life, I know what it's like to almost lose everything, so where I'm at now is no big deal. I'm chasing my dreams and have a great life and I fought like hell to be where I am.

Chapter 17

CHEMOTHERAPY OR RADIATION TREATMENT

"You have to be willing to give up the life you planned, and instead, greet the life that is waiting for you."
- Joseph Campbell

Now with each chemotherapy treatment I always feel a little different, depending upon the drug therapy I am on. Different treatments have different side effects. Some side effects happen after every chemotherapy treatment. I always get itchy during the first week or two until the chemicals gets out of my system. I am very exhausted the first couple days, which makes training much more difficult. I work extra hard to push myself along with it. I always sleep more a day or two after as well. After chemo, I walk out of the hospital feeling fatigued. I have had so much chemo that I have learned to get my training in as fast as possible after I get home. I have generally scheduled myself for the hospital's first appointment in the morning. This gives me a routine where I wake up early to get treatment by 8:00 a.m.

The drug I'm on now I seem to be handling the best of any so far. A few years ago I was on a different drug and I had the worst side effects.

One time when I was on this drug, I was itching so bad that I went to the hospital up the street and just stripped out of all my clothes. Yup, I was butt naked. My doctors think it's because the trial drug I was on before combined with the treatment I'm on now stayed in my system for about a year. I would throw up, couldn't wear clothes, had constant fevers and pain everywhere. Even my ears were hurting. The headaches, nausea, and constipation were constant and unbearable.

My current drug regimen is administered once a month. I get to the hospital at 7:00 a.m., get my blood work to make sure everything's okay, and get approved for the treatment. Sometimes if my test result levels are bad, I don't get approval for the treatment. Cancer seems to have a mind of its own and it tries to out-think the treatment, which it knows is attacking it. Cancer is a savvy adversary.

I've had over 10 drugs and God knows how many trials I've been on. Before first trying a new drug I got pretty nervous. I'm thinking about how many times they are going to stick me with the IV. Usually, it takes anywhere between two to five times to get the IV in my hand right. Are there going to be side effects? Will they be different, the same, more intense?

When I first was diagnosed you would think I would be really nervous. But to be honest it wasn't till I lost my hair that it really hit me that I was sick and could die. When I had the first treatment, I was fine for the first few hours afterward. But later in the night, I remember my dad putting blankets on me because I was shaking like crazy and had a bad fever. So, after the mouth sores, the nausea, the pain in my bones, sleepless nights from chemo, I always think, *What if something goes wrong and I'm never completely okay?* Chemo is a tough thing to deal with. I've had chemotherapies that lasted for days or some that last for eight hours. The quick chemotherapies (under two hours) I know wouldn't hurt me too bad so I left the hospital fine. Once you get to hour four, you just feel really bad and it just gets worse. Especially for the first few years I had such strong drugs my counts would get lower and when that happens you just feel like crap. Because all of these things happen, I always feel like this. It's almost like what one of my brothers says: "I'm going to punch you in the face but I'm not going to tell you when." So, you constantly are thinking, *When is it going to happen; when am I going to suffer?* When I get nervous before the chemo, I always am okay with the nurses leaving the room because during those couple minutes before I get the IV, I try to enjoy the silence and stay calm because you never know what could happen. Once the drip starts anything can happen and you don't know if you are going to die or some kind of emergency can happen. I've gone to chemotherapies where the person next to me passes out. I have seen a person suffer a stroke. There is nothing I can do to help because I am getting my treatment next to them. Even if I could, how would I know what to do? My "go-to" reminder and mindset companion is to take off my ring and look at the "FEARLESS" inscription, or I merely rub it and just remind myself to be strong. I have to if I want to stay alive and live to fight another day.

I think it's important when you are going through treatment to have certain mechanisms to help you deal with such a mature challenge and struggle. It has to be real and raw. No Superman costume. The battle is real. I call on my faith and hold on to personal mental and physical mechanisms to survive and just get myself through the next day. When I get home and I know the treatment was strong, I pray to God for strength and for him to look over me while the drugs do their job.

The worse thing is when you go through the toughest chemotherapies and you literally can't imagine how the cancer could be there after all that, and then you get a scan and find out it's worse. There's nothing more defeating than this conversation with doctors. It's like the monster in the video games that keeps coming back even after you hit it with all your weapons. Relentless. And when that happens you think to yourself while you are getting the chemo, *Am I wasting my time? Is this even going to work?* But you remain positive, in spite of everything. I've been blessed that I've never had a chemotherapy treatment where I was alone. My mom and dad have been to every treatment and I get to talk to them, which keeps my mind off of what is going on. See, I'm the kind of person whose mind is in constant motion, always thinking. For me it's just natural to go to the what ifs. But as the years go on, I get stronger and stronger mentally. I know I have to do treatment for the rest of my life. As long as I am on treatment, I know I am alive and fighting. I'm happy I'm on a treatment right now that doesn't make my life so miserable. So many years I would look at the bag filled with chemo and go, "Can't wait to be jacked up." I would say it not to be negative, it was just something to joke about. Anyone going through cancer treatment knows it's normal to be upset or nervous. My dad told me something before my first chemo that I will never forget. He said, "Anthony, do you want to live? Do you want to lose?" And I looked at battling cancer as if I was an athlete and I want to win the championship, which is beating cancer. Some of my battles took multiple different chemotherapies and multiple years to beat it. I am a winner, not a whiner.

When I go into treatment now, I put on my music, bring myself a bottle of water, and talk to my mom. I try to joke around, which gets my mind off of it. And sometimes I'm pretty tired because I like to wake up extra early, sometimes around 4:30 a.m., so I can do my cardio and watch some TV. There's something about waking up and going straight to treatment that just bothers me. To me getting up early and going through a routine before treatment says I started my day off by building my strength and then having a planned time to relax. The day starts with me being productive, which takes the anger away. I've done this so many times I've accepted it, but it's not something I like to do. That's why I'm so happy it's just once a month.

Now I've had over 100 radiation treatments and to me I'd rather do that than chemo. I'm in my underwear in a cold room and it lasts for about 5-10 minutes, then I get to go home. Most of my radiation treatments are every day and continue for two weeks. One treatment went for four weeks but because it's done so quickly, I didn't really mind it. I never get nervous before it and half the time I'm asleep so it doesn't really bother me. The big negative of the radiation is that it has caused permanent damage to my hip and back. I have tons of scar tissue near both parts. At one point in my battle, I had a 13-cm mass in my hip. Picture something the size of an orange in your hip. That caused a lot of problems and to this day training is very painful but I push through it. Now the chemo caused damage but not damage where I need to take pain meds. So, the difference is with chemo my mind goes everywhere or it did when I first was doing it. But during radiation, it doesn't really bother me at the time, but afterward I pay the price by feeling quite a bit of a pain. To this day I'm still suffering from the damage of all my treatments. So yes, while I'm sitting on a freezing table practically naked, I think about what this is going to do to me in the future but at the same time I have to do it. I was told once or twice that if I don't do the treatment, I will go through tough things like being paralyzed in one leg or paralyzed in both legs. Hearing stuff like that is hard to deal with just because you are afraid this will happen to you. With the hip, months after the radiation, I was so nervous when I walked because I thought the cancer would take the feeling away from my legs and steal my mobility. But while on the radiation table, I keep telling myself it's going to work, it's going to work, because I've been blessed that it has worked every time and I have the most amazing doctor. So, when he tells me I don't have a choice, I just go with it and I really do trust him completely. If I had the choice, though, I would choose getting chemo over radiation just because even though going through it makes you suffer way more, it hasn't caused me permanent damage physically. I've gotten better at dealing with all these things. I am proud of the fight within me. I have had supporters help me stay positive and confident that the fight does and will pay off. I don't even think about the chemo a couple days before or even a week before. I just wake up, get my business done and move on. It's part of my life now and will be for the rest of it. I know that may sound sad but I'm very strong and I wouldn't be that way if

I didn't go through the things I've been through. I remind myself of that and thank God for all of it because I'm proud of how I have gone through everything. I'm proud of the people I've helped because of it.

If you are going through treatment, just know it's okay to be nervous. It's okay to be constantly thinking of it. Just know you can get through it and keep telling yourself you will keep fighting until all the treatment is done. During one treatment, I told myself literally over and over for four straight hours, "I can do this, I can do this. You are stronger than the chemo. You can do this, you can do this." Telling myself things helps me get through tough times. I know it made sound stupid but telling myself things over and over helps me believe in myself and makes me stronger.

Chapter 18

RELATIONSHIP WITH MY BROTHERS

"My greatest gift from my parents was giving me my brothers."

I have two younger brothers, Vincent and Michael. It was tough for them when I got sick and I knew they took it hard. My entire life I was always the one looking after both of them. No matter what, I was always there. I can't tell you how many fights I got in protecting or defending my brother Vincent. I was raised as the oldest to always look after them, no matter what. And even if they were wrong, I still would be on their side. To be honest, I never really had to defend Michael because everyone liked him and he didn't have a big mouth. Now I'm not saying Vincent has a big mouth, but he never stepped down from anyone and that caused me a lot of trouble. Even when Vincent and I were playing hockey, if anyone did something that either hurt Vincent or did something I didn't like, I would always take the person out. I love my brothers more than anything and I would take a bullet for them, no matter what.

Growing up, my brothers and I did everything together. Whether it was playing roller hockey every day, relaxing with video games, playing basketball or any type of sport you can think of, we did everything together. Even though we aren't the same age we hung out with the same friends, especially Vincent and me. To this day all our friends hang out together and we are closer than ever. We tell each other everything and we always have each other's backs. It's amazing having brothers like that.

When I got sick, I think my youngest brother Michael took it the hardest. I never saw him cry, but I could just feel that he was afraid and it hurt him to see me suffer. Now personally, I only think there were a few times where they thought I was going to die. My brothers can easily take care of themselves so I'm not saying they need me in every sense. But we are so close we tell each other everything. For the people out here who are also the oldest sibling, you can understand where I'm coming from when you feel like you need to always be there so they don't have to be in pain or get nervous or fearful. It's tough having that responsibility, but it's something I was raised to do. I will be looking out for them for the rest of my life.

My favorite time of the day is when my brothers are done working and we are in my room watching TV shows or movies. It sounds kind of weird but the older we get, the closer we seem to grow. I can't imagine my life without them. When I first got sick, my first thought was, *What am I going to do? I can't die. I have to be here for my brothers.* I was more concerned about how they would take it than anything else. I never saw them cry but I could see how much it was hurting them to see me sick. I went from always being there for them to needing them to help take care of me. For the first time, the roles were reversed. When I was diagnosed, my brother and I were attending Fordham University and my youngest brother was in high school. Vincent, every weekend, would come down from our apartment and spend time with me. What he didn't know was how much that meant to me. He would work and study all week and instead of partying he would come down from the city to hang out with me. Even if I was with my girlfriend and if my parents were there, he would still come just to try to be there for me like I was there for him my entire life. It was tough when I first lost all my hair because it was then I knew I was very sick and this whole thing was very serious. I'm sure that was the moment when it hit my brothers as well because they could see the physical signs of how sick I was. No matter what I needed, whether it was picking something up from the store, or renting a movie, or even making me a sandwich, they tried their best along with my parents to be there for me in every way. One of the things out of all these years that I was most scared of or one of the top reasons for my intense fight was the following question: "What would happen if I died and my brothers lost their older brother?" My family always has something going on and we all have to be around to help and pitch in.

Two years before I was diagnosed, I was in the car with my girlfriend when my mom called. She was so upset because something happened to Michael. They thought Michael might have cancer. I saw in my mom's eyes how scared she was. When she told me I remember I just stopped and prayed with my girlfriend in the car. I begged God if someone in our family had to battle cancer, to please let me be the one who has to be sick. Later, I remember literally begging in the bathroom where I was praying, *Please let it be me who gets sick.* It's ironic that a year or two later I was the one who got sick. I thought of that moment and told God, "Thank you that it was me." I said, "Bring it!" I looked at cancer as a competition. I looked at it as there was no way I was going to lose and everyone who knows me knows I hate losing and I don't lose.

So as the years have gone by, I have kept fighting and each time pushed back cancer. Vincent graduated from Fordham and Michael went to Stevens Institute of Technology in Hoboken, New Jersey, which is a great engineering school. I was very proud of my brother for getting in there because he worked so hard in school. I always told him to stay at school and that he didn't have to come home to be with me. Now he still came home but not as much as Vincent did while in college. All the years I was battling cancer, all I could think was, *I can't let my family down.* I had to beat this thing. I truly believe that my taking care of myself the way I did made a big difference in why I am alive. I boxed for almost five years and I think my brothers were proud I was a boxer, especially while I was sick.

More importantly, I think it made them feel that I wasn't going to die. When I needed to find a donor match and when we decided to make a documentary about my fight, my brother Vincent was right by my side. He is an actor and he is also a talented photographer. So, as we worked on the film, we found two great filmmakers and Vincent was there for every day of shooting. He would pick out my clothes, he would do my hair and other things to help. When the documentary was released, I did so many interviews. My brother never missed one interview. He knows how hard it was for me to conduct so many interviews but we needed to find the donor match and we needed to inspire people to sign up to be tested and enter the donor registry that would help other people in my position. Vincent was always there; he would drive to the city for doctor's appointments or chemo if my dad had a business trip.

When it came to being donors for a stem cell transplant, my brothers were a perfect match for each other but not for me. I understood but, to be honest, that really sucked. To Michael, it didn't matter that he wasn't a perfect match. We decided to go forward with the transplant because it would give me the best chance of survival, and Michael volunteered to donate. So, he took all the shots and did everything he needed to do in order to raise his counts and prepare himself to donate. During this time Vincent moved out to California and lived with my good friend Katharina Harf who is the CEO/President of the great Foundation committed to cure blood cancer, called DKMS. He was living there to chase his dream to become an actor and at this point he had management and all that. After my 30 days in the hospital for the transplant, Vincent left everything he was working on in California to be there for my parents and me. The first day he was there, I was in the hospital room being irrigated for eight straight hours because my bladder was bleeding. I was in so much pain, I screamed begging to be put out. I'd scream, pass out, scream, then pass out and that went on for eight hours. For the next seven months every day was the worst day of my life and my brother helped my mom with everything. Whether it was getting blood work, getting a check-up, getting me to my appointments and procedures, he was there. I will owe him for the rest of my life. My parents aren't the only reason I'm alive. Both my brothers committed to me and my fight. Having such a loving family meant all I had to do was look at them. One look and I knew I had to fight. I couldn't let them down and when I didn't want to fight for myself because of the unbearable suffering, all I had to do was look at them and I knew I had to keep fighting harder and harder.

The transplant from my brother Michael didn't work, but I still have a feeling his cells changed my body and that's why a lot of different treatments have worked over the years. Now my doctors don't agree with that but my mother and I have this weird feeling about it. Doctors can't always explain things that seem to not have a medical or scientific explanation. The funny thing is I used to pick on my brother Michael for his partial red hair. Before the transplant my beard was blond and brown. Now, after the transplant, my beard has turned red. Talk about karma; every time I see my beard, I think, *Wow, payback time! This kid gave me red hair.* What a turn of events and some humor that we must all find during times like this.

When I started getting really sick, which happened when the cancer came back after the transplant, I knew my brothers were scared. They had every right to be. I just kept getting worse and worse. But soon after, when I found out I had beaten brain and blood cancer, there was such a relief for all of us. When I learned of this huge win against the cancer, I was alone for the first time in the doctor's office. Most appointments I was with a family member but this time my uncle became sick. My father had gone to see him. He called me and said to come to the hospital and say goodbye to Uncle Steven because Dad had a bad feeling he wouldn't make it. So that joy I got from my miracle quickly left because I was so afraid I'd lose my uncle. After

I said goodbye to Uncle Steven, my brother drove me home. But of course we can't plan how life deals us unforeseen events. Sometimes it feels like when something amazing happens, there can be a setback or something bad/sad happens shortly after. Maybe this is life's way of telling us to stay grateful and humble. So when I saw my uncle, he asked me how the scan went and I couldn't be the one to tell him because he was so sick, but he forced it out of me and I told Uncle Steven my cancer was gone and he smiled then closed his eyes.

All I wanted to do was go home but a 25-minute drive turned into 13 hours because the George Washington bridge was closed. So, I got my miracle but I was stuck in snowstorm traffic and I was worried about my uncle.

Still, once at home I immediately told my brothers about my miracle and their eyes were full of joy and relief. We all celebrated the next day.

I never tried to vent or show pain to my brothers, but when I suffered from the pain or the panic attacks or from setbacks, they would see it and I would feel guilty. This is another reason why I train so hard. I wanted my brothers to see me being strong. I want them to know I will never leave them and I will be there for them when they get married, when they have kids, when they get a house. They will never be alone because I will be there for them. I thank God every day for keeping me here so I not only can help other people but I can be there for my family.

Chapter 19

STRONGMAN TRAINING AND WHAT IT DID FOR ME

"Every time I got stronger, even if it was just by a pound, it made me feel that much farther from death."

While I was battling cancer, it was attacking my entire body, including my brain. At one point when I was the weakest, I stood six-feet one-inch tall and weighed only 141 pounds. I remember all my clothes were baggy. My shirts felt like dresses, even my underwear wouldn't stay up. I was eating only once or twice a week. My first memory of being in the hospital was actually at that point when I was getting better but I didn't know it yet. For eight months of my life I have no memory of what was going on. I laid in bed all day, every day. My last memory was of breaking up with my girlfriend. Fast forward eight months and I weighed 141 pounds and was barely able to walk into the hospital bathroom.

My mom found a way for me to stay in a lavish hospital room for my treatments. Remember, this was MY first memory in eight months. What am I doing here? I learned that Mom fought for me every day. Because of how hard she fought, I was able to get access to this room for my family and me. Eight months is a long time. There were times when the hospital wanted to move me but she would have none of that. My family in no way could afford that room; hell, not many people can afford any of this kind of medical care. But my point is that the room really became a second home to not just me but to my family. I remember once when my family was in my room talking. They were talking about all the weird crazy things I did in those eight months and looked back on how bad things were. My youngest brother Michael made a joke saying, "Remember when you took a swing at Dad? That was so funny!" I didn't remember, and in no way, shape or form would I ever lay a finger on my parents. So when I heard I'd taken a swing at Dad, I wanted to go to the bathroom and cry because I felt so bad. But because I was so weak, I couldn't walk to the bathroom so I broke down in front of everyone. It was that moment I knew I needed a change and I needed to get my strength back. So, while I was still in the hospital, I looked up workouts I could do in my bed. At this point I couldn't complete a single push-up, let alone one pull up. While I was searching on Instagram, I saw something I used to watch when I was a kid on ESPN. It was a strongman competition. I thought it was the coolest thing. These guys were pulling 18 wheelers, flipping thousand-pound tires, deadlifting cars and more.

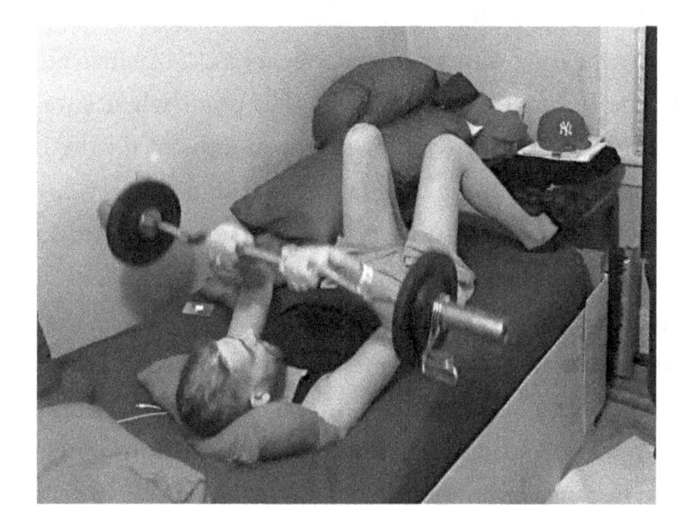

When I got home from the hospital, I knew I wasn't ready to do anything like that. So, my brother would bring circling bars to do skull crushers in bed. He'd bring dumbbells for me to do dumbbell and overhead presses. Every day my brother Vincent would hand me weights and I'd have a weight-gainer shake right after I did these exercises. I knew I couldn't box anymore because I couldn't get hit in the head after having my brain filled with cancer.

I had two "no-quit" objectives once I got home from the hospital. I needed to beat cancer, which had anchored 47 lesions all over my body and had my filled my brain completely. Next I needed to get as big and strong as humanly possible. Day after day I would work out in my bed. After about two weeks, I was able to do bodyweight workouts including push-ups and pull-ups. I'd be on my knees for up to an hour trying to do as many push-ups as I could. Every day, I would try and do more and more. During this time my uncle moved into our home while he was battling his cancer. He thought I was so crazy working out in my bed and on the floor. But I remember telling him I'm going to be a monster, you'll see. I'm going to be as big and strong as possible. I knew my health was getting better because I kept getting stronger and stronger. I even gained a little bit of weight. I told myself once I could do 25 push-ups, 5 pull-ups, and 30-lb dumbbell presses, I would find a gym that can teach me strength training even if I was in a wheelchair. My uncle was so proud of me. This pushed me to the point where I would get three days of chemo, then I would work out in the hospital and work out when I came home. I remember one day I had a puke bucket next to me on the floor and I turned on strongman videos on my TV and I kept telling myself I'm going to be like that. And after I was doing my push-ups, I would puke, do more push-ups, then puke and repeat.

After Uncle Steven passed away, I told myself I needed to be strong. So the next week I took my wheelchair and went to strongman gyms to train. But just like with boxing, I was told that once I got healthier I could be trained. Now I was familiar with this disappointing feeling, but I was more motivated than ever to find someone to train me. Now I did the first thing I needed to accomplish. Then I received my next miracle; I beat cancer for the fifth time. While I was on my way to the third gym (after getting a "NO" from the first two stops), I was praying in the car that the gym owner would say "YES" and teach me/ train me. I got out of the car with my wheelchair. Music was blasting inside the gym and it made me a little anxious but I was ready to do what I needed to do. The guy's name was Frank and he recommended I take the classes. I told him classes were not for me. I wanted to do strongman training. He was a young guy but I remember him saying, "Hell yeah, I'll train you. It's badass you want to be a strongman after beating cancer for the fifth time."

At that time I weighed 141 pounds. I was using a wheelchair but I would get up and do the exercises. Frank gave me the workout plan to follow and each day I got stronger and stronger. Now the problem was just because I beat cancer didn't mean I didn't feel like I was going to die. And the thing that removed the fear of dying was to see myself getting bigger and stronger. So, some days I would throw the weights if I wasn't stronger from the day before. Something I need for everyone to understand was that I needed to see and feel progress. You see, being a cancer patient taught me that cancer never quits and any day that I don't see progress gives me the feeling that cancer just gained a day on me. That was unacceptable. When I saw and felt progress, I truly believed that I was keeping my distance from the cancer gaining on me. Every pound of weight I gained, every pound my overhead log press went up, every time I lifted a heavier stone, I felt farther from death.

Strongman training is the scariest, hardest, most fulfilling training I've ever done. There was a time I was walking the yoke machine with 700 pounds on my back. I completely went from a cripple to a stronger, healthier person and it was because of the strongman training. In 13 months, I went from 141 pounds to 230 pounds. I wasn't fat, I wasn't bloated, I just ate everything I could find. I drank my shakes and I turned into what I was obsessed about, which was being very big and strong. None of my jeans fit anymore and my shirts were tight. And that's exactly what I wanted. I trained so hard to feel strong and to be strong.

During this time, I still had chemo every single month. Every other week for eight months, I would get chemo. Yes, the cancer came back, and when it did, I didn't miss a workout. When my cancer came back, I needed radiation on my spine. I was still setting personal records (upping my workout achievements) in the gym. These results gave me the confidence to know if I could do that, I wasn't going to die and I wasn't going anywhere.

After my radiation was over, my best friend bought a ticket for me to travel to the Cayman Islands. I was so grateful because I had never left the country before. Even though I was in so much pain on the trip I was just so grateful to be there. My brother Michael went as well. For that trip I was willing to put my strongman training on hold. I only missed training that one time in over 13 months. Once I got back home, I continued with the training. I was also accepted into a clinical trial in North Carolina that could potentially cure my cancer. I was in North Carolina for three weeks. This trial had many potential side effects. My mind and body were strong and I was confident that nothing could take me out. First thing I did when I got to North Carolina? Yup, I found a gym and got a membership.

The chemo was pretty strong for this trial, but after treatment I'd do my strongman training at the gym. I couldn't do everything because they didn't have all the equipment, but I improvised and didn't miss a workout. Unfortunately, the trial didn't work but my training never stopped. The point of my explaining all of this is that strongman training gave me strength and hope that I would survive, just like boxing did. I'm always in pain and when I train the pain is even worse, but I always push myself. I'm always trying to better myself in every way possible. Strongman training not only helped me physically but it made me even stronger mentally. Strongman training was the hardest training I've ever done in my life and it was even harder because of how sick I was.

When I'm really sick, I can't do anything physically. For example, when I had a bad case of pneumonia, I couldn't go up even half a flight of stairs. So, my point is when I do these things physically and I accomplish them, it eases my fear and anxiety. I know I can and will fight anything. For those out there afraid they are going to die, take up some physical activity and try to get better at it, whatever it is. The better you get the more confidence you will have and you might even tell yourself, "Holy crap, how did I do this if I'm so sick!" It means your body hasn't given up on you, so you shouldn't give up on it either.

I was at a gala a few years ago. It was held to raise money for blood cancer research. I met a man with his son and he told me how much he admired me and my story, so I took him aside and we spoke for a few minutes away from the crowds. I knew his kid was sick so I wanted to try and help anyway I could. His son was a rower and the dad was saying because he's sick, he shouldn't row any more. I told him to do the opposite and the best feeling in the world will be when you beat the person rowing next to you while you are getting chemotherapy and he isn't. Little wins, added up, lead to the confidence that you can handle anything that comes your way. I told him I didn't listen to everything my doctors said. This was especially true when it came to building my strength. Physical exercise during the treatments that really made me tired and fatigued gave me the confidence to keep pushing and fighting. Yes, it was hard but it gave me so much mental confidence that the next treatment, while difficult, could not beat me.

I believe doing things physically helps us survive. I found out months later, this young kid from the gala was one of the best rowers on his team. I learned how great he felt beating the other kids while he was sick. I also learned that he beat cancer! The father called me and thanked me for that conversation. The kid went back to rowing, he trained hard and he fought hard, and he beat his cancer. I can't tell you how much joy the phone call from the dad brought me. Just because you are sick doesn't mean you can't accomplish things. Just like boxing and the strongman training—it didn't just help me survive, it made me strong mentally. I know I can face any challenge when my mind is strong.

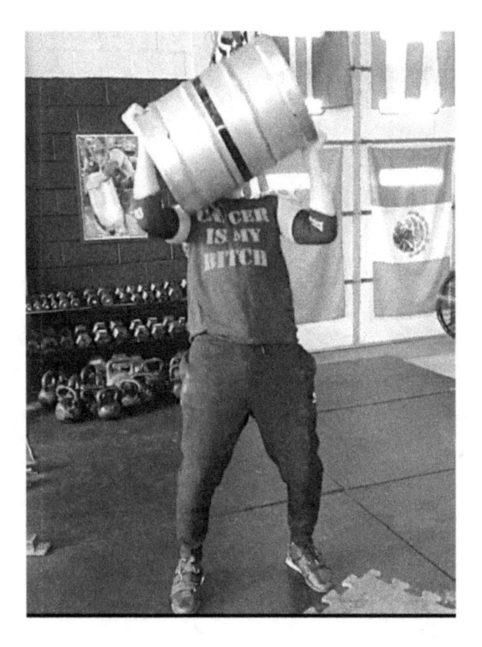

Chapter 20

MY BROTHER VINCENT

"I looked after you my entire life. But you chose to look after me. It was seeing you every day that made me fight harder. Without you the story would've ended a long time ago. Love you, bro."

IN VINCENT'S OWN WORDS:

"Daily doctor's visits, weekly hospital trips, and treatment monitoring. Where is the light at the end of the tunnel? Nobody prepares you for this. Nobody could ever have prepared you for this. Confront every battle head-on and don't worry about what's next until you're done. Take everything that comes your way week to week and tell yourself a fresh start is only days away." Those words were repeated in my head multiple times a day. That thought process started as a day-to-day mentality and eventually evolved into an hour-to-hour, minute-to-minute and sometimes even second-to-second mindset.

Putting words to paper has never been a challenge for me. I've written screenplays and research papers, and have had my work published, but this is different. Standing tall and confronting what my family has gone through for the past decade is no small order.

Where to start? How to start? Which details are too big and what stories are insignificant? The truth is that nothing is insignificant. When you completely consume yourself with one goal, everything outside of that begins to fade away. Whether you're a professional athlete, a student, or a newly hired employee at a company that nobody has ever heard of, the same thing happens. Goals are set and those who want to achieve them do everything in their power to make it happen. Again, this past decade is no different. My family and I set a goal even though all the odds were stacked against us. We weren't out there to prove anything to anyone. The only thing that was on our mind was our goal. From day one to the present time, our goal was to keep my brother Anthony alive.

My brothers and I were always very close with one other. Anthony and I saw much more of each other simply because we are fourteen months apart as opposed to Michael being three years younger. Anthony always experienced things first, from high school to sports and even dating (if you can believe that). Unfortunately, if one of the three of us was destined to face such an illness, he was chosen first. I'll never forget the feeling of when my eyes truly opened up to what my family and I had actually been doing for so many years. It was after Anthony was in remission for a third time and that period lasted the longest. It took a handful of years, but this looked like the real deal. Nerves were calmed and just as life started to seem to balance out, Anthony's scan results came back. My family and I had been rolling with the punches for so long that when news came back that his cancer had shown up again, it hit us like a freight train. The ability to relax was almost the worst thing that could've happened to us, in my opinion. It was in that state that everything we all had personally been dealing with, especially me, was truly being digested and understood. What our daily routines had been for so many years prior finally came to light because we thought that the light at the end of the tunnel had finally been reached.

Among many things, Anthony's illness has taught me to go after what you want in this world. Futures aren't known or guaranteed to anybody. For so many years I experienced living in finite periods of time, which made planning for anything recreational extremely difficult.

Cancer is an illness that can easily be thrown around because of the sheer amount of people that are affected by it. Learning about Anthony's illness opened up a world that I never thought I'd see. Cancer really opened my eyes up to what people in the present and past have gone through. It's almost as though if you haven't been around the illness that you don't really understand what it's like. There were too many instances where my comprehension for what was happening every day had become my very existence. Many people say that their family is close; I believe ours was always great too, but there's nothing like staring death in the face every day for a decade to really show you how much your people mean to you. It's very easy to say that Anthony was destined to be in the position he's in currently with the platform that has been created because of his struggles, but that would be a fallacy. My older brother has clawed and sometimes crawled his way to get to where he is now. I believe it was Confucius who said, "It does not matter how slowly you go as long as you do not stop."

Anthony, from being inside the eye of the hurricane I can confidently say that because you did not stop, you have achieved one of your goals. You have beaten the odds and went twelve rounds with Death himself. Now it's time to pat yourself on the back and conquer your next goal. I hope you don't worry about me. Because of you I couldn't be prouder of the man I am today. Just because you were sick doesn't mean that you weren't the greatest big brother I could have ever had. I know that this is only the start for you and I can't freaking wait to see what wall you knock down next. You're my hero, Anthony.

Chapter 21

AFTERMATH OF BRAIN CANCER

"It's hard to beat a person who never gives up."
- Babe Ruth

The weird thing about brain cancer was that something happened that never happened in all the years I was battling the other cancers. I experienced a thing called "chemo brain." This is where I became forgetful and couldn't focus or concentrate the way I could before the cancer. I would say every person I've ever talked to that has gotten chemotherapy has gotten "chemo brain." It was very difficult for me when I was at Fordham because I would study all night and then I'd wake up and I wouldn't remember a thing. The fact I had a 3.1 - 3.3 GPA in the three semesters I was there was a miracle in its own right. The hardest part of "chemo brain" was that I had to compete for grades with what seemed like one hand tied behind my back. This made me angry. I worked harder than I thought I needed to work. This work earned me a 92 average and I ended up with a B- grade, but hey, that's just how it was. It was very frustrating over the years when I'd be having a conversation and I wouldn't know what the hell I was talking about. Now honestly, I was upset about it the first year but I chose to make jokes about it. This seemed to not only make me feel better but the people around me felt better too. All the speeches I've ever done or during the interviews I've given, I've avoided having any chemo moments. The fog of "chemo brain" comes out of nowhere and more often when I am relaxing. I am fortunate.

I told you about the eight months for which I have no memories. When I started to realize what was going on around me, I was confused. I thought I still had a girlfriend, I thought I was still boxing, I thought I was bigger. In reality, no relationship, no boxing, and I was quite thin and very weak. There were so many things I didn't remember. Not only were those eight months gone, but I also couldn't remember some of the high points of my growing up years. Not remembering these milestones really scared me. It's hard to admit it, but I was terrified.

I was fighting for my life and I questioned what the point of living was if nothing good ever happened to me or for me. The only positive was having my brothers and parents by my side at the hospital. While that is a huge positive, all my friends stopped talking to me for whatever reason, the girl I was in love with stopped talking to me, and it was almost like I had to find a reason to fight. All the years I fought I always knew things would get better. This is the positive mindset that I held on to. All the people I inspired or gave hope to over the years, I had no recollection of those conversations or phone calls or discussions. I remember being in the hospital and going on to my social media. That is where I learned so much about my life and experiences I had. Crazy, right? Everyone knows how Instagram works—you post a photo and then a description. I had photos of me boxing, my interviews, the things I did with friends and family and even though I would read the posts, I had no memory of these events or what they were like. The good thing, even though I didn't know it at the time, is that my brain cancer wasn't so bad as it might have been. Eventually most of my memory has returned, but at the time I really didn't know what was going on.

When you are too weak to take care of yourself, it is very easy to get scared. I didn't want to die but there were times when I didn't know if I would wake up the next morning. It is also very difficult to comprehend anything beyond the next day. I was so weak and so sick I couldn't even take care of myself because of how weak I was. The first couple weeks I really was scared because I didn't know what was going on and I obviously didn't want to die. But there was a part of me that thought maybe it would be better if I did die so that I wouldn't be in so much pain and so that my parents wouldn't worry anymore, wouldn't have to care for me, and could get back to a normal life. I thought my life was one constant fight, one unstoppable bout with pain. Besides my family, I didn't know what to hold onto. Crazy, right? I didn't realize how tightly my parents were holding on to me.

But as the days went on, I started to get better. I began remembering things like my first hockey game. I scored two goals in my first hockey game when I was a kid. I remembered vacations with my family and how much fun we had. I remembered how it felt when I got into Fordham. All those years my teachers didn't think I would go to a good school and that I wasn't smart enough. I remembered the feeling of getting in and why I wanted to go there—so I could be a lawyer and help people. Little by little I started to become myself again, which took about a year. Once I started working out in my bed and my sick uncle came and lived with us, he helped me a lot uncovering the person I was before the brain cancer took over. I didn't really talk to my old friends, so my uncle became my best friend, along with my brothers.

The whole process was very scary. Just imagine going to bed one night and you wake up in the hospital eight months later. You don't remember anything good and you're hooked up to all these machines pumping cancer-fighting treatment through your body. I could barely walk. I remember looking at my legs and I was freaked out because all the training muscle development was gone. The only place I felt safe was in my room. I was having panic attacks constantly, though I realized I had to keep fighting because I couldn't have a mental breakdown and lose it. This made me very scared. I did begin to remember clearly all the people I spoke with and how I was trying to help them. I couldn't let them down, but the scary part was that even while my mind said keep fighting, I wasn't always sure how to do that. I really couldn't take care of myself. I had to get help walking to the bathroom. I needed help changing my clothes. Dinner was brought to me. Sometimes I had trouble getting out of bed and making it to the bathroom. My bed was only five feet from the bathroom.

Again, when I wanted to get my strength back, my brother would bring up dumbbells and weights and hand them to me in my bed. During my entire battle with cancer, I was never at a lower point than I was with the brain cancer. I felt like I was a mental vegetable and I couldn't find my way out of it. Honestly the worst part about the whole thing was going to bed at night. I never really spoke about it to my family but I was terrified of going to sleep because I didn't know if I would wake up. What ended up happening was I was getting night terrors every night. And in each dream, I ended up dying and often with very frightening images of how. Too often the image was of being in a hospital bed with tubes down my throat. I barely could breathe and I ended up dying that way. I did NOT want to die that way.

Right before I died in my dreams, I would wake up in a pool of sweat. I did a pretty good job over the years dealing with fear. With the brain cancer, however, I had a very hard time dealing with it. All I kept thinking was, I have to get better; I have to get stronger. Even if I didn't remember many good things, I would beat this thing and make sure I lived to make the most amazing memories. That's the point I got to. Hell, if I couldn't remember good things, I was going to make good things happen after I beat this cancer. Every day my goal was to make good memories and get stronger, no matter what I had to do.

When I woke up and my memory started to return, it took about six weeks for me to feel significantly better. I was motivated to make great things happen. I was going to appreciate and be grateful for them. Any memory I could recall or new one I could make was gold. Maybe it was when Uncle Steven and I talked and laughed for a couple hours. Or maybe it was a meeting where I was helped someone deal with being diagnosed with cancer. Getting stronger physically and the feeling of lifting something heavier. Stepping on the scale and seeing how I was gaining good weight and wasn't so small and skinny any longer. I could keep going on and on and on about all the things I tried doing and remembering. But during this time when something good would happen there were also bad things happening as well.

The biggest example was my miracle happening in which I beat cancer for the fifth time and then my uncle died a month later. Other examples would include getting a good scan then getting really sick for the rest of the week. But I realized life is always this way, that there had always been good times and setbacks even before the cancer. For instance, getting into the college where I was going to play hockey, then getting hit by a car a week later. So I changed what I wanted to do with my life and got into Fordham. Then, I had a severe itch for months and had vertigo for two months in my first semester. It's simple to say, "Stay positive. You can do this." But it's something I really had to deal with over the years. I can easily give over 100 examples of what I just explained. But to be honest, everything I've been through has only made me stronger. I truly believe our hardships are what helps us become stronger. It's okay to be afraid, it's okay to question yourself, it's all completely normal. So many negative things have happened to me as I'm sure have happened to everyone else. It's all about how we roll when hit by a setback.

When I was a kid, I wish I'd known that our hardships help us grow. It would've been a lot easier to deal with things; it's part of the process of growing up. I hate that I'm even saying this but an example is when my manager gives me a call and gives me some good news, I find that a "what could go wrong?" question is still in the back of my head. So I've learned that bad things happen, and I work to embrace it and even to say, "Bring it!" I've learned not to back down in my life.

In battling cancer, in my career, in my family life, I refuse to allow the fear of something bad happening to control my life. To be honest, it did control me for the first couple years I battled cancer. I was trying to be an athlete, and I wanted to raise awareness for cancer and for people that need transplants. At the same time, I was trying to give people hope and strength. The fear took some of the joy away from the things I did and I wish I didn't let it because it affected my life for some time.

I tell myself I'm going to do whatever is required to achieve my goals and stay healthy and if setbacks happen, then they happen. You can't allow fear to take over. If it does, it's important to learn to embrace it and deal with it when it happens. That is all that matters. Trying to be fearless is something I strive to be. But I still deal with fear in my everyday life. I deal with the fear of having a panic attack, the fear of dying, and the fear of failing, which is my biggest fear. I don't do well with failing in whatever I put my mind to. I hate to lose. Whether striving for great things or dealing with a disease, I'll fight for the rest of my life. Whatever bad happens I'll deal with it and move on. These days I don't dwell on the negatives. I take a step back and evaluate the situation and see what I need to do to get past it.

Cancer is stressful. It affects everyone who loves and cares for you. As the person struggling and battling a disease that can take my life, I've learned that trying to be happy and strong helps the people around you while you are going through it. Now you can say, "It's all about me. Why should I worry about the people around me when I'm the one suffering and going through it?"

The reason is that thinking about others and not just yourself makes you stronger. It forces you not to feel bad for yourself and ultimately when you do beat the disease, you'll be happier that you did it with the help of others AND that you worked your tail off to win. There's nobody in this world in my opinion who doesn't want to be strong. When life gives me an obstacle, I say, "Bring it." Yes, it hurts. Yes, I feel fear sometimes, but knowing in the end I'll be stronger makes me feel like I can do anything.

Beating cancer five times has made me feel like I can do anything because of how difficult it really was. Unfortunately, now that the cancer has returned, there's no cure for me but I don't feel sorry for myself and I don't want anyone to feel bad for me. I'm learning how to enjoy every good thing that happens in my life. I am 100% about finding the good stuff. I wasted so many years not enjoying the challenge of beating cancer and many of my other accomplishments along the way because I was waiting for the next bad thing. Those days are gone!

I remember I flew to California to do a scene in *A Star is Born* with Bradley Cooper. Now I'm no actor by any means. My brother is the actor in the family. But once we finished filming, I stayed in California for a few days. Upon my return home, I got a lung infection and ended up in the hospital. While I was in the hospital, I completely forgot about the coolest thing I did just a couple days earlier. I forgot that I was an actor for a few days.

Yes, it's understandable because I had was attached to an oxygen tank and fighting the infection. But I wish I didn't let the infection take over the joy of the movie experience. I regret that. I knew I wasn't going to die even though I literally couldn't breathe without the oxygen tank. But still, these days, every time I experience something positive, I try my hardest to be in the moment and enjoy it. Why waste a second thinking about what might happen to me? At one point in my life, something good happened to me, then it was like I had a gun in the back of my head and I didn't know when the trigger might be pulled. That's no way to live.

I really believe in staying positive and doing what makes you happiest, no matter what it is. Cancer can be a great (but insanely difficult) teacher.

Life can be hard and sometimes it will bring you to your knees and keep you there if you let it. That is one of my favorite lines from a Rocky movie. It's a favorite because it is the truth. We don't know how much time we have, so my point is to try and do everything you've always wanted to do and stay positive during tough times. Yes, you definitely have heard that before but it's the God's honest truth. When you accomplish something, embrace it.

When something bad happens take a step back and get yourself through it because you can. I'm living proof of that. People have told me plenty of times I'm going to die and not only were they wrong but I'm doing better than I ever have in my life and I'm enjoying everything I do in my life and I stay positive about my cancer. If it gets worse, I'll beat it again. I know it, I believe it. Even though I know I'm feeling better than I ever have in the past 12 years, it doesn't mean I don't still have problems. I have had a great deal of trauma inflicted on my body from all the chemotherapy and radiation.

Knowing that every month for the rest of my life I have to go to the hospital to get treatment is a really tough thing to deal with. It was tough and still is tough mentally to stay strong and positive. Every time I feel chest pain or I have shortness of breath, my mind immediately says, "Is it the cancer? Is my body getting worse? Am I going to die? Is this the beginning of the end for me?" All these things cross my mind every time I feel something like that. In reality, it could just be heartburn or indigestion. That is the hardest mental challenge to conquer and not let it take over my head. I work hard to just let it go but sometimes when I wake up in crazy pain it's so hard not to go down the path and say to myself, This is it. I used to let it take over so many days of my life. I wasted those days in allowing my cancer to control my life.

On top of all the problems when things were good, they were great. I wish I didn't let so many memories get ruined over the fear of being really sick again. I would go on dates, or I would be at an event speaking, or I'd be having a great interview, and I would let one of those pains take over the joy of it.

So, it took me a long time to be able to just let it go and truly live in the moment. I'm so happy I never gave up because I really do love my life. Some people might say, "How can he love his life? He's going to be battling cancer for as long as he lives. He has to do physical therapy for a long time. He's in pain every time he works out. It's hard for him to put shoes on." But the reality is, if I'm breathing, you can't count me out. Every time something good happens—whether it's for my career, a good workout, or just not feeling pain—I embrace life and love every second of it. Like right now I'm in pain writing this but I don't care because I'm writing a book! This is something I've always wanted to do, and I'm not allowing my pain or the fact my cancer might get any worse to take the joy of that from me.

Chapter 22

MY RELATIONSHIPS

"The few relationships I've had during my cancer battle were blessings. Even though my life was never easy, those I loved were always there. We experienced life together outside a hospital or a bed. We drove one another crazy. But loved even harder."

Now, ever since the age of fifteen, I've been dating. I'm the kind of guy that likes having a girlfriend and I've been blessed to have had a few amazing relationships, even when battling cancer. The two times I was in love, I was battling cancer. There are so many people out there with disabilities or who are sick with cancer who think they can't find love. All the girls I've been with are absolutely amazing. When I first was sick, I remember I took a nap and I woke up with a ton of hair all over my pillow. That was a really hard moment for me because I really was insecure. They say it's way harder for women to lose their and it's probably true but it was really hard for me. I thought to myself after I lost my eyebrows, *What girl is going to want to date me? I look like Mr. Clean, for crying out loud!* All I needed to do was put on a white shirt and I'd look the part, except for the muscles. I learned to deal with it. I thought to myself, *I'm at war right now with my body and losing my hair is proof I'm fighting for my life.* I embraced it as a badge of honor almost. I remember the first girl I was dating told me, "Anthony, I don't care that you lost your hair. You are just so confident and so strong, that's all I care about."

Now, a lot of people, including my family, offered to shave their heads too, even my mom, but I told them no, I didn't want them to lose their hair because they weren't battling for their lives. I treated it like a scar. I'm going to beat this thing and make a full comeback.

It is tough dealing with relationships when you are so sick. My heart broke every time I got a scan and it went wrong. I knew not only would my family be upset but I also needed to comfort my girlfriend, saying, "Don't worry, I'll get through this." I've had so many scans that were bad and it wasn't my family I would worry about because they didn't break down. They didn't show fear. Now obviously they were dealing with fear, but I felt it was my responsibility to give my girlfriends hope. Well, some deal with it better than others. I mean, I loved them and I didn't want them to be in pain. I really did feel guilty. All the kids my age were graduating from college and traveling the world and I was in the hospital all the time. With every girl I dated while I was sick, I would always feel guilty. I would go out though because obviously a girlfriend doesn't want to spend all their time shut in and not going out. But again, like every other potential setback, I used having a girlfriend as a reason to get out of the house. This cancer thing wasn't going to hold me back.

It was a double-edged sword. You're in love and you have an amazing relationship. But at the same time, you have to push yourself to do things because you think to yourself, *Not only am I sick but what girl is going to want to be with someone that doesn't leave the house?* I can't tell you how many times I was at a bar and I would go to the bathroom, throw up, and put some gum in my mouth and pretend nothing happened at all. It used to stress me out because I really did try to be a great boyfriend. And yes, dating was a great distraction from the cancer, but I always felt guilty and I would put a 100% effort into my relationships, no matter what.

I was raised to be a good guy and that's what I was. The worst part about having girlfriends is when the relationship ends. Just like anyone else you get depressed and you get sad. But at the same time, you are really sick and you have to fight for your life. Boxing really helped with this. Not only was I in the gym for hours but it really helped me get over a relationship. It was just the hardest on the days you are really hurting and you are so sick you can't get out of bed so not only are you thinking about, *Am I going to die?* But you are also thinking about how much you miss the person you were with and how you feel alone. Even though I was never alone because of my family, I couldn't have many distractions because of how sick I was. When it was great it was great, but when it was bad, man, it was really bad.

The thing I did with every girlfriend, especially when I was cancer-free and when my cancer came back, I would say, "This is a really hard thing to deal with, and if you don't want to deal with it, we can break up." Yes, I was always so nervous they would take me up on the offer, but I was lucky enough that with the relationships I had, most girls stayed with me.

It's hard when you are sick and at my age everyone was finding out who they were and they were able to do so many things. As for me, all I thought about was how I was going to beat cancer. Then I would think, *I have to live. I can't just stay in bed all day.* I tried to have as normal of a life as I could. I was an athlete, I was involved in charities to help people, I would go out and travel and I did a lot of amazing things so I wasn't just in bed.

The cancer left me and everyone always on edge and everyone was always afraid. Many times I had to tell my girlfriends, "I'm gonna make it. I'm gonna do it." It just sucks to see the person you love hurt so much for something that isn't anyone's fault. I would get upset that the girl would be hurt seeing me in pain or going through treatment.

There was nothing I could do. I am just grateful for the relationships I had because of all the good memories we created.

Now after the brain cancer, I forgot all those memories. Eventually many of those memories came back to me, but still it sucked to forget some of those special times and have to be told about them instead of remembering them for myself. There are great times to this day I still don't really remember even though I've been told about them, but it's for the best and I don't dwell on it. One day I'll remember it all, I tell myself, because it's just how it is. It's in the past and it's time to move forward.

Chapter 23

HOW I AM IN HOSPITALS

"Once I take my first step into the hospital it reminds me of my story. The good, the bad, the ugly. But even though it's mostly pain, I walk in proud because I'm still here."

Being in the hospital is stressful and I think this is probably true for everyone. With as much time as I have been in the hospital, these days I am much less stressed and not scared. It's where I go for my treatment. They know me there.

When I first was diagnosed I can't tell you how hard it was to be strong and just to go in for treatment without being upset. I remember the first chemotherapy treatment I had. I didn't complain but I was nervous. I just sat there with my parents and listened to music. A big reason why I was scared and nervous was because a couple weeks before treatment, I did my presentation in my college communication class about cancer. I researched cancer for months. I thought to myself, *When am I going to lose my hair? Am I going to be able to leave my house and have a life? Will I be able to do well in school and graduate?* And the biggest question: *Am I going to DIE?*

It's very stressful and really depressing in the waiting room. You see people who are so young and so old that are so sick and it just scares you. For people who don't have cancer and don't go into hospitals very often, it's a hard thing to deal with. When you see people who are sicker than you, all you can think is, *Am I next? Will that happen to me? Will I be in a wheelchair? Will I be hooked up to an oxygen tank?* All these things have passed through my mind over the years. The worst part about it all is you get to a point when you just want to get it over with and leave. There are so many times when my scheduled appointment would be pushed back. This is hard to deal with. Just picture yourself doing something that you are so nervous about and you just wait, not knowing when you will be called and you just want to get it over with.

As the years went by, I would always get nervous. My family and I live in northern New Jersey and we go to New York City to see my doctors to get treatment and tests. My dad has always driven me to doctor's appointments. These days I ask him not to but it's nice that both my parents are so involved. My point of saying this is that when we would get to the George Washington Bridge, I would start getting really nervous because I knew it was just another thing I had to deal with. I've had about 1,000 hours of chemotherapy and over 100 radiation treatments. Each time I go over that bridge, I think to myself, *It's game on*. I treat it these days as a sport. I get in the hospital and I have to win. Now you may be asking yourself, "What does he means by that?" The way I win is that I don't get emotional. I don't get scared. I see my doctor and am ready to receive my treatments and walk out of there alive.

Every time I walk out, whether I'm sick from the treatment or not, it is a win. If I don't leave the hospital because I'm sick or something happened, I lose. It gets pretty boring there so I try to stay occupied, whether that is watching a movie on my phone or listening to some pump-up music. Now you may think I'm crazy when I say this, but I listen to heavy metal music just like I do when I train to get me pumped up and ready to go. Covid affected my routine because I was only able to bring in one person and that person is always my mom. I always feel bad because my dad isn't allowed in. He just sits in the car for hours and when we are finished, he drives us home. Now I know I'm so lucky to have both of my parents there for everything. I've talked to many people who have gone into treatment by themselves and I always felt so bad for them. It makes me feel amazing because I have such a great support system and team. Years ago, when Dad was often on business trips, my brother Vincent and Mom would drive me. Because the chemotherapy was so strong over the years, I couldn't drive myself home because it would be dangerous.

Sometimes I go to the hospital and get great news, but most of the time over the years I would get bad news. The first time I was ever told I was going to die was after the second transplant. I was in the hospital and that was so hard to deal with. I immediately stormed out of the room and went to the bathroom. Hearing that you're going to die when you are only 25 years old is a hard thing to deal with. I had fought so hard for so many years. I just couldn't believe that after being in Texas getting treatment for eight months, now they were telling me the treatment had failed and now there was no cure for me. How is it even possible my cancer could come back?

While in Texas, I almost lost my bladder; I was so weak and I was getting blood transfusions every single day for months. Every day was the worst day of my life in Texas. Literally each day sucked more than the day before. I would wake up and consider the day before and think, *Wow, that was the worst day of my life*. And then that day would be even worse and so on. So, hearing this news from the doctor was something that broke my heart.

After spending a moment in the bathroom, I went back to the exam room with a motivation like I have never felt before to prove the doctor wrong. My dad asked how much time I had. Because it was spring, Dad asked, "How about Christmas?" And the doctor said, "Christmas is far away from now." The doctor was telling us I didn't have much time. Mind you, Dad is the toughest man I've ever met. He was a Ranger in the Army and I never saw him break down. When I looked at him after the doctor's comment, I saw tears running down his face. All I wanted to do was stay strong and prove everyone who doubted me wrong.

Now, you may be asking, "What about your mom? How did she react?" My mom is one tough cookie and when anything bad is about to happen in her life she steps up and you can see it in her face. She said, "Not my son, not my boy. You'll see he's stronger than you think." Now the point of my telling you this is every time I'm in the hospital, I think about that day. It was one of the worst days of my life and even with the brain cancer I never forgot that day or that moment. I try to tell everyone I speak with that they will get stressed in hospitals or have doctor's visits that are tough.

We are so fortunate these days we can listen to any music we want on our phones; we can watch movies and all that. Currently I'm writing all of this in the hospital and it takes some of the stress away. I will have to be getting treatment for the rest of my life and that's something I very much take seriously but I try to find ways to be happy instead of being scared or anxious. It's tough for me and it will always be tough for me to be in the hospital because there are just so many people who are so sick. I don't want people to ever feel bad for me or to pity me. I take it as an insult, to be honest. The hospital taught me how to step up and get the job done. I've learned how to be strong and get after it. The reality is, yes, treatment sucks but I'm here to get better. I'm here to beat cancer again and every treatment I get brings me closer to that. For those going through cancer, try and think about that. It gets worse before it gets better, but I know if I keep fighting it will continue to get better over time.

The worst part of the hospitals for me are: 1) staying overnight and not being able to go home, and 2) getting biopsies and undergoing procedures. Let's talk about not being able to go home. One of the reasons for overnight stays is a procedure like cell transplants. The first transplant was when my cancer came back the second time and they used my own cells to strengthen my immune system so it could fight cancer on its own. Normally people are in the hospital for about 10-17 days for this kind of treatment. That was tough for me because I was very uncomfortable. Anyone who has stayed in the hospital overnight knows the food sucks and the beds are uncomfortable. Just lying there will put you in pain. I also felt bad because my parents would sleep in chairs. You would think you'd be able to sleep in the hospital but that's not the case. The nurses wake you up every 4-6 hours to check your vitals and draw your blood. So honestly, it's just very annoying and what sucks is the people around you could be doing better or are near death and you constantly think to yourself, *Am I going to be like that? Am I going to die?*

The first transplant really opened up my eyes to what actually could happen. During my first transplant I would lock myself in the bathroom and work out just because I wanted to prove I was going to win again. Remember, my mindset was that if I could work out, then I was not dying. Exercising was probably stupid because I had an IV in, but I would do push-ups and pull-ups and ab work. It kept me strong physically and mentally even though I was going through chemo. It was the first time I was really stuck in the hospital and when I would try to sleep, my chemo pump would beep every five seconds and it kept us all up. It was hard not to think of the worst because you feel like you are in a place you don't want to be.

When I got chemotherapy treatment for the transplant, I had my first-ever panic attack. I remember I was eating a toasted bun with jelly and all of a sudden, my chest got really tight, I got shortness of breath, and I lost all feeling in my hands. At that moment I thought I was going to die because I had never been through anything like that. Now, I got out of the hospital as quickly as possible during my transplant. I looked at it like a competition, just to motivate myself mentally to get this thing done. To help me stay strong mentally and to avoid panic attacks, whenever I have a stay in the hospital, I take time to work out. I really do believe it helps me through the hospitalization and helps me recover faster. I've been in trouble when I got caught working out, but to me it's worth it.

You have to do whatever it is that helps you make it through. It's just so hard not to think of death and to remain positive when you are going through something like cancer treatments. Nurses are constantly coming into your room. A team of doctors comes in every morning and it just feels like you are truly in a bad spot. It's also hard because you have your friends texting you and they are either traveling, playing sports, or even partying and you are just stuck in the hospital. I really did suffer mentally in the hospital but at the same time, it helped me grow up and appreciate life and for that I am forever grateful.

The same thing went on during the second transplant except I had a lot of problems. I had a procedure near my heart because I had so much fluid in my chest. I almost lost my bladder and I had a handful of procedures done with that. With every biopsy and procedure, if I had the choice, I wanted to be awake for it. It's probably a control thing, but every time I sign that waiver, I always feel like there's a chance something could go wrong and I won't wake up. To this day I still have trouble with it. I'd rather suffer in pain than be knocked out no matter how bad it is. In 2020, during a biopsy procedure, I felt like that was it. I even wrote 32 letters to the people I care most about. I really thought I was going to go and I wanted those people to have something from me in case I didn't make it. I ended up having a procedure where they had to take a tissue biopsy from my lungs to find out what kind of pneumonia I had. That was at least my 30th biopsy and procedure. You would think it would get easier but it never does. I just pray to God during those times and ask God for strength and if it's my time please look after my family like they've looked out for me. After every biopsy I am always in pain. Whether it was a spinal tap, a bone marrow biopsy, or taking samples of my cancer at any point in my body. Staying in the hospital overnight always sucks for me and the worst time is for biopsies. Unless you've been constantly awakened by nurses, have had trouble breathing, or been in for serious pneumonia, you may not understand how bad staying in the hospital really sucks. I was in the hospital for six days during a biopsy and I think it's the waiting that is the worst.

While you are in your room you are just waiting for the worst to happen because at the end of the day only God knows what will happen and all you can do is lean on your faith. I pray a lot in the hospital, which isn't something I did at first when I was battling cancer. My faith has gotten strong over the years and it's helped me get through a lot of tough spots. Praying in the bathroom in the hospital makes me feel so much better. It makes me feel like I have an angel on my shoulder and it not only gives me confidence but it takes a lot of anxiety away as well.

The thing about hospitals is when you are in there anything can happen. I've had regular doctor appointments where I was supposed to go in and talk to my doctor and I ended up being admitted five minutes later. The most stressful visits were in my first couple years of battling cancer where I'd get a scan and instead of calling me and telling me the results over the phone, they asked me to come in. When we got the call to come in and meet with the doctor, I immediately thought the worst, because what else could I be thinking? It's human nature to be negative in that sense but over the years, I've trained myself to remain positive every time I'm in the hospital. Now sometimes you get yourself all worked up and in reality nothing is wrong. But because you have had so much negative happen to you, I think it's just normal to be fearful. For those people who are battling cancer, going into the hospital being positive really does make the difference. A big reason is that when you are positive you take the bad news even better and it's less of a heartbreak.

Every time I go to the hospital, I always think to myself that I was told I have no cure and that I might not make it to the end of the year. I don't think of it as being negative because that was five years ago and I'm doing better than ever. I hope for the best and prepare myself for the worst. The worst things that have happened to me have been in the hospital. I remember there was this one day they pushed back my chemotherapy later in the day so my parents and I were just sitting there in the waiting room. I saw so many people sick in so much pain and it was just a reality check. And that day I had chemotherapy and the IV was put in my arm. I had a reaction from the chemo where my arm literally blew up and the veins were black. I was in so much pain and all I could think was, *How am I going to box after this?* Instead of thinking about what chemo they would put me on next, all I could think about was how I was going to box when I couldn't even lift my arm. My arm got so big it grew about four inches thicker with black veins. It was one of the freakiest things I dealt with. But I was able to think about something I loved. Instead of thinking about living and not dying, I thought about boxing. And I think everyone that is battling something needs to have something so important to them like that. It makes you stronger and being in the hospital unfortunately sucks up everything. It makes you scared, it makes you tired, it makes you anxious, it never leaves you especially once you have had something bad happen to you.

Once the bad thing happens, it leaves you scarred, and it's up to you to leave it where it belongs and that's in the past. That's a life lesson I learned from being in the hospital. Instead of dwelling on the what if's and worrying about the next thing that might to happen, you have to look forward and focus on the things you love, and if something happens you deal with it and move on. I've had to be strong with every visit I've had. I would say 90% of my doctor appointments have been negative: "Anthony, your hemoglobin is low so you need blood." "Anthony, your platelet count is low so you need platelets." Platelets and blood were very important to me for boxing. Having a low hemoglobin level leaves you taking five steps and you can't breathe. So, imagine that with boxing I had 50% lung functioning and with a low hemoglobin I couldn't breathe so it made boxing so hard.

The other reason why it affects boxing is platelets stop you from bleeding out. It clots your blood so it will stop bleeding. I could go on and on about how this level was too high and this level was too low with almost every organ in my body. And as a 20-something year old you think to yourself, *I'm so young, how is this possible?* And what they don't tell you is most doctors give you the bad news and walk out of the room so you're left feeling awful. I'm blessed to have found a doctor who really does care about me and not only makes me feel better but my family as well. And for those reading this and are battling cancer, take it from someone who's beaten cancer five times over a 12-year period. It's not about having the best doctor; it's about having the best doctor for you and everyone else that's battling alongside you. That's something I learned in the hospital. Every time you have an appointment, ask every question you possibly can and never leave the room without knowing everything.

When I first was battling cancer, my parents would ask all the questions but I didn't ask mine because I was so focused on the chemotherapy or radiation I was going to get. So many times, I left the hospital depressed and so stressed out it really affected my life in a negative way. It would ruin the rest of the week for me and that really sucked but I learned to open my mouth and say what I needed to say.

Now the other scariest thing I've dealt with in the hospital was when I needed radiation. Mind you, I have had over 100 treatments. I'm lucky enough to have a world-renowned radiologist who also knows how to talk to me. I was told so many times that if I don't get radiation, I will be paralyzed. I will lose feeling in my leg or legs. I would be in a wheelchair and all that nonsense.

The part that bothers me most is the prep for radiation. I laid on the table one time completely naked while they gave me a scan and then gave me tattoos. Now I've been to a tattoo parlor and these tattoos feel way worse than the tattoo I got probably because they dip the needle in ink then stab you basically in the weirdest areas. I have more than 50 blue dots on my body just with radiation tattoos. One time for fun with one of my ex's, we played connect the dots with them before my radiation treatment. The real funny thing was I forgot to wash the ink off so when I went into the room the guy saw it and we had a nice laugh. It just always sucks because you have so many people in the room making a cast for you and you are literally sitting there for an hour. But honestly radiation only lasts for a few minutes each time and never really makes me sick but it gives me permanent nerve damage and that's why I'm doing physical therapy and probably will for a long time. I'm fortunate enough that radiation has always worked for me but honestly even though the radiation is easier to handle at the moment, down the road it has been worse than the chemotherapy and that is why I preferred chemo over radiation. Besides being told I'm going to die by my oncologist, the radiation appointments were scarier in a different way because hearing you won't be able to walk again is a tough thing to deal with and I've heard it a handful of times. So, on the way home from hearing that it was really hard. And when it got hard, I would pray to God for strength because that's something that's made me feel a hell of a lot better because my faith is strong. Every time I have my head down in the hospital more than likely I'm praying because I know God will get me through this.

The most stressful time besides the second transplant was going to the hospital during Covid. Both my parents have been to each and every treatment I've ever had. My mom had to fight just to get in and be with me due to the restrictions of Covid. So, what happens is we get there by 7:00 a.m. and get blood work and wait for the treatment to be ready. Luckily the treatment is short but my dad is just stuck in the car the whole time and I always felt bad about that. The good thing was my hospital has another facility 15 minutes from my house. When you get there, they take your temperature. Then they ask you all the Covid questions. Then they make sure you have a mask on. So many precautions. What sucked the most was I was so worried about getting Covid because they say I'm high risk because of all the treatment I had. It made me feel like if I contracted Covid, that would be it for me.

Luckily I can do all my work at home, but going to the hospital made me fearful because of how serious this thing really is. I wouldn't go on dates; I wouldn't go to the gym; I worked out in my garage. I didn't see my friends and that was all at the beginning of the pandemic.

You could tell that everyone in the hospital was so afraid. Six feet apart from everyone. Having to wear a mask. And God forbid you took your mask off to wipe your nose or you'd have someone that works there be on you in a second to put it back on. I remember I was in the waiting room along with everyone else and somebody coughed. I swear all 30 people whipped their heads around so fast to look at the poor person. The environment in itself was just so scary and stressful. And then you had to get treatment on top of it. All everyone wanted to do was go home and be safe.

Luckily, I would do telehealth calls instead of having to see my oncologist. Now I love my oncologist but no way did I want to go to into New York City, especially because of how many people were sick there. The hardest part for me was what happened to a new friend of mine. His name was Dave and he was having a tough time in his life. His wife left him and he had no family near him, so he reached out to me for advice about his cancer. Now over the 12 years I've battled cancer, I've had quite a few people reach out and I am so blessed because I've had the opportunity to help in a small or big way. Anyway, Dave and I were getting closer and he was a good guy and I was trying to help him—whether that was trying to lift his spirits or telling him what to do about side effects, or just generally encouraging him. Unfortunately though, he passed away a couple months into the Covid pandemic. And it wasn't the cancer that took his life. It was Covid. Now, we are talking about a strong, young, in-shape guy getting through the chemotherapy pretty well, but once he got Covid that was it. He contracted it while he was in the hospital and it really sucked that he passed away. God rest his soul.

Because Dave got Covid in the hospital, it took a while for me not to get nervous about getting it too. Now I always believed I would survive it but only God knows when it's your time and that really hit me after that happened. He wasn't my best friend but he was a good dude and I was proud to call him my friend. It took almost a year for me not to get nervous about Covid in the hospital and it was something I just had to deal with. It's a reminder that life is so precious and try to live every day like it's your last. That experience reminded me of that and that's why I stopped getting nervous in the hospital. Whether it's about chemotherapy, radiation, a lung infection, just anything that could happen, you have to remain positive and stay strong no matter what situation you're in.

Chapter 24

CANCER AND WHAT I LEARNED FROM IT

"It's through our greatest sufferings that
God shows us our greatest gifts."

Cancer is something we all know about and it has probably affected you in one way or another. Whether it was you personally or it was a friend, a family member, a wife, or a husband. Cancer is a very serious thing and it has taken the lives of millions of people worldwide. Now for me, if I'm being honest, it's made me suffer in more ways than I thought were possible. Whether it was physical, emotional, or even spiritual, cancer has affected me in all areas of life. Even so, for almost 12 years I've battled it tooth and nail and I don't regret a thing. This is the battle I am facing now with the cards that life has dealt me.

If I was asked, "Anthony, would you, if you had the chance, have it all taken away and have what people call a normal life?" the answer would be no. Now obviously part of me wishes it didn't happen because of what it did to my loved ones and the people who care most about me. The stress that it has put them through is something I will always feel guilty about but the reality is it's not my fault and nobody should feel guilty for having an illness. In fact, cancer has taught me a great deal and changed my life in positive ways.

First of all, cancer has taught me the importance of faith. I always believed in God my entire life but it was through my journey where my faith really took another turn for the best. I'm not the kind of person that shoves my faith in God down people's throats but I do tell people how much strength God has given me. My faith makes me feel like my journey is for a reason. A big reason why I tell my story is because I know it helps people. And by helping people it makes me feel as though my family and I were meant to go through this and there was a higher reason for all of it. On a powerful note, what doesn't kill you makes you stronger. Every time I'm going through something, whether it's a problem with my health or something going on with my family or people I'm close to, I turn to God and, to be honest, it makes me feel powerful.

That's not to say I haven't struggled when it comes to faith. When I first was sick, I was so mad at God. I thought he took hockey from me and now he's taking my life from me. When I was first sick my girlfriend at the time thought it would be a good idea for me to go to a priest to try and make me feel better. All the priest said to me is that there's nothing God can do to help you. All that will happen is you will live or you will die. It was so upsetting hearing that. I knew he wasn't going to say God would cure me so don't worry, but I didn't expect him to be so negative. For a time it turned me away from God. But through my journey I turned back to God and I am forever grateful for everything I have been given.

When I was a teenager, I was having a tough time with school, friends, hockey, family, and all that. I felt as though I was weak mentally and that's why I couldn't get through those things in a good way. I asked God, "I don't care what you have to put me through. I don't care how hard it is. Please help me be as strong as humanly possible." Now, I didn't ask for physical strength, I asked for strength emotionally, mentally, and everything in between. I'm such a different person now than I was then, and to be honest, I'm so proud of the person I've become. I've made a difference in this life and I hope God gives me the opportunity to help people even more.

When was there a time in your life where all you could do was fight? To be honest, even though dying was always passing through my head I always tried to fight. I never let thoughts of death take over and allow me to stay in bed all day and be sad. I chose to force myself to stay strong mentally. I was raised on the belief that what's between the ears controls it all. Obviously meaning the brain. I had to force myself to believe I'll survive in everything I did. Every time I had chemo, I would tell myself in my head over and over, *This is going to work, this chemo is going to kill my cancer.*

I always felt like I had God looking out for me. I told myself there was a reason for this and I need to get through it so I can help people, which is my true passion. It's hard to explain what it's like when you are slowly dying. You feel like your soul is slowly leaving you and it's such a scary process. I would see people not taking care of themselves health-wise, not taking care of themselves by smoking a cigarette or not exercising. That bothered me so much because I would do anything to be healthy. Every day, my heart broke and all I could do was fight. The way I fought was through prayer and exercise. I had to believe God had a higher purpose for me and that helped me a lot. At the very least it gave me the strength to go out gracefully.

Cancer has taught me how to live in the moment and to appreciate all the good things in life. In these 12 years cancer has done so much for me on a positive note. It has helped me grow up. It has helped me have the confidence to be able to get through anything in my life. It has taught me that miracles do happen and you can be that person who experiences a miracle. It has taught me how to be so strong that nothing can keep you down. It has helped me appreciate every day like it was my last and to live in the moment. I think about small things, like watching a movie with my brother and laughing, or playing with my dog. There are so many examples but I think it's most important to live in those moments and to appreciate them whether they be good or bad, as long as you learned from them. Cancer has taught me how to be strong when it counts.

Yes, cancer played a role in a lot of physical damage to my body. I have scar tissue all over my body. It damaged all my veins, either because I was stuck so many times with needles or because the chemo was so strong it literally burned my veins away. I walk with a limp because I had a 13-cm mass in my hip and the radiation caused so much scar tissue damage it feels like a bone when you touch it. I can't feel my toes because of how bad my neuropathy is from all the chemotherapy I've had. I'm on pain meds because without it I'd be in severe pain every day. I take over 30+ pills every day whether it's for my thyroid, neuropathy, pain, anxiety, and of course my vitamins. Some nights I wake up in so much pain. I have a cane next to my bed to help me get up and move around at random times in the night because of all the damage my body has gone through. In addition to the physical toll is the mental and emotional toll. I have PTSD and it's very difficult for me to sleep at night because of the night terrors I get. In each night terror I dream of dying and I wake up huffing and puffing because of how bad the dream was. I get panic attacks almost every day and they can happen when I'm laughing or I'm working or I'm training. They happen at random times during the day. The point of saying all these things is because for someone reading this you might say to yourself, *This guy's life is miserable. His life sucks.* That's just not true. It's been hard, yes. But no matter how many problems I have, I love my life and I just appreciate the fact that I'm breathing.

Cancer helped me really focus on what I do have and to truly live in the moment and to enjoy it all. I don't stress about my cancer growing and my having to change treatments. I don't focus on how I'm in pain all the time from all the damage my treatments have done to me. If I focused on all the negative things, I would be the most miserable person on the planet. I think that's important for everyone to do in their lives, which is focusing on what we do have in times that are bad. What are the things you do have?

What cancer taught me was how to adapt and how to love life and take charge of what's in my control. Every day I'm doing things that I love, which is helping people. Whether it's an interview, a call to help someone battling cancer, having a speaking gig, planning things for my Foundation, the list goes on and on and I thank God every day for everything he has done for me. Cancer didn't just teach me how to be strong and survive. It taught me how to appreciate life every moment, the good and the bad.

Cancer has taught me how to get through the toughest moments in my life. There's nothing I've been through tougher than dealing with the fact that you feel like you are dying. And when you are told you basically will die of cancer, it makes it way worse. For me that's all I could think about the first time I was told I would die. All I could picture was my dad, who is a tough guy. He doesn't show emotion and when the doctor said, "Christmas is far away," implying I wouldn't live that long, there were tears running down his face. I saw that and knew I had to fight in spite of what my doctor said.

Keeping your head on straight when you are told you are going to die after fighting so hard for so many years is heartbreaking. It affects every part of your life. Your relationships with friends or a girlfriend. It affects your family because they are scared. Keeping yourself strong is so hard and was the hardest thing I ever had to do because it was an every-second-of-the-day battle. Sometimes I would ask myself, *Should I stop treatment and give up?* I've thought maybe I'd just stop treatment and do all the things I've wanted to do, like packing up and traveling to see the Northern Lights. That's always been one of my dreams. But stopping treatment to do those things would mean giving up. And I couldn't give up, I couldn't lose, and that's how I looked at it. I did everything. I did holistic treatment, I fixed my diet, I did trials for drugs. Everything I did was so I could survive. It's hard to live your life and go about your day when you don't know if this will be your last day alive.

Focus on getting through your challenge, whatever it is, by thinking of the things that are good. When I get down on myself, which everyone does, I like to think about how far I've come and what I do have. The great thing about it is everyone can do it. It took me a while to be able to do this, especially when I thought I was dying. I felt as though I had nothing but, in reality, I always had something. I like to believe everyone has at least one good thing in their life. Now it's hard to imagine anybody who doesn't have at least one thing, whether it be good health, family, friends, going to college, or traveling. There are so many things people have done that have brought joy to themselves. I learned to focus on those good things while I was battling my disease. What are some of the things in your life you appreciate?

My focus is on my family. Yes, we may be crazy but we love the hell out of each other. During my hardest days, they were the ones who got me out of bed and got me to take the needle for chemo. They were the ones who got me out of bed to train to make my body strong so that I could survive and beat cancer. The reason why I'm saying this is to express what cancer has taught me. How to go through hell and come out the other side an overall better person. With all those problems I have I'm a happy, confident person. It made me a better person. Someone who would help anyone and would take the shirt off their back to give to someone if they needed it more than I do. It's all about how you perceive things. Before cancer I wasn't happy like I am now. I didn't take all the medicine I take now. I didn't do chemo every month. I didn't have night terror every week. I didn't wake up in massive pain every night. And yet I wasn't as satisfied with life as I am now. The difference is I appreciate my life and I soak up every second doing the things I love and being around amazing people who inspire me.

Cancer taught me how to be more compassionate. It has helped me be a better person, a more compassionate person, a more empathetic person. A person who listens to people and really cares, because helping others is my passion. The joy I feel for making a difference, no matter how small or big, is what life is about for me. Cancer has taught me to be honest with myself instead of lying to myself. It has taught me to believe that everything and anything is possible regardless of the odds. It has taught me to love others unconditionally no matter how much they have hurt me. Cancer did not ruin my life. It took many things from me but it didn't take my life from me. Everything I do every day I'm passionate about and I love everything I do. It's made me strong and refined. It taught me how to be more empathetic to whatever someone is going through no matter how big or small the situation is. It helped me find out what I really want to do with my life which is helping people. After I broke my leg and my hockey career ended, I never thought I'd find something that brought me so much joy.

Telling my story so I could find a match was what first gave me the opportunity to help others. I started inspiring others just from how I was battling cancer and the things I was doing and it made me feel like I was making a difference. So many people tried helping me by swabbing to become bone marrow donors to remove my blood cancer. It made me feel so good that my cancer wasn't just affecting everyone in a negative way but also in a positive way. I haven't yet found my perfect match, but because I shared my story, so many other people got perfect matches and have gotten transplants so that they could beat cancer and move on with their lives.

Cancer taught me how to take a risk. When I decided to take up boxing after the first time my cancer came back, I got rejected by coaches and people didn't want to fight me because I was sick. But I kept trying until I found a coach who would train with me, and later on I got respect from the people in the gym so they would fight me. I couldn't tell my doctors that I wanted to box because they were horrified by the thought of me being in the gym, let alone fighting people.

I pursued boxing anyway because it was what I wanted to do, and through doing that I started to develop a lot of confidence.

After battling cancer the first time, I could barely get out of bed. What I learned was how to take my medicine a certain way and eat or drink whatever I had to do to get myself in the gym and train. I took risks in my life but not something like this. I was so sick, but by going to the gym I was doing what everyone else did and that made me happy. It taught me that anything is possible. Imagine your sickest day with all the ailments I had and still leaving your house and going to fight. I knew that by taking the risk, I could end up in the hospital and I could be in even more pain. But I did it anyway because when I did, I not only felt like an athlete again, but I felt like a person again. Not just some person in the hospital all day who didn't do anything.

Cancer showed me in the beginning years that anything can happen. Nobody has the right to tell you that you can't do this or you can't do that. When I was young, the teachers would say I wouldn't be able to be like the regular kids. Basically, they made me feel like I wouldn't amount to anything. So, to show them wrong, I got fantastic grades and went to an amazing school. That was before I was sick. While I was sick, I was told I couldn't do anything because I'd be too sick. And that was my biggest fear—that I'd be in a bed all day throwing up or rushing to the bathroom and I wouldn't have a life. Now there were times in my journey I really didn't have a life and I didn't live life to the fullest. That was why I finally decided I wanted to be a risk-taker.

Every time I worked out, whether weightlifting or boxing, I would tell myself I was getting stronger and I would get myself all amped up to perform better even if it was after chemo. And to be honest, most of the time I was weaker. But I would tell myself, even though at times I could barely breathe, *I'm going to win. I'm going to win. I have to win, this is it.* A lot of times I lost but I kept telling myself, *I can do this.* I tried being better at everything in my life.

I tried my best to be better at everything and there were periods where everything was worse but I started to realize that the more I kept telling myself, I can do this, I started to believe I wouldn't die. I must've told myself a million times, *I can do this, I can win, I can do this, I can do this.* I started believing in myself and when that happened, I was getting better. After I was told I was going to die, all I kept thinking was I wanted to beat cancer to prove that doctor wrong. Have you ever been doubted by someone you trusted? I experienced this from someone I believed in and he looked at me as if I was a statistic and that motivated me in ways I can't even describe. I thought about it every day. Those words echoed in my thoughts and strengthened my faith. When my miracle happened and I beat brain cancer and the cancer all around my body, all I wanted to do was tell this doctor that he had been wrong about me. Nobody should be judged; anything can happen and I'm living proof of that. That was more than five years ago and I'm doing great.

Cancer taught me to believe in myself in every aspect of my life. I needed to believe in myself or I would've died. Cancer is such a hard thing to deal with and the reality is you can't escape it. You can't just push the pause button on being sick. Or being in pain. Or getting panic attacks. Cancer is a 24/7 job. In my life before cancer if I was having a hard time, I would find a way to escape to get my head on straight. But with cancer you can't do that. You have to deal with it every second. Everyone is so afraid of dying it's depressing and overwhelming. It taught me to believe in myself and to be positive with everything. A scan, chemo, radiation, or even getting bad news from the doctor. You have to be positive or it'll suck all of the energy out of you and leave you feeling lost.

Before the cancer, I first learned to believe in myself when I was on the ice playing hockey. The sport meant so much to me and when I scored, I believed I could do it again and again and again. It simplified in my brain the whole concept of the sport and the job I had to do. Get the puck and put it in the net. That was so easy for me to be able to think that way. Still, there were times in my hockey career when I had trouble believing in myself. When I would try out for really good teams, I would doubt myself because of how good everyone was. But the reality was once I got on the ice, I knew what I had to do and I would end up making the teams anyway. So, when I got cancer, I tried thinking about it the same way: don't overcomplicate the situation, just simplify it.

So I started off trying to tell myself to get up, go to the hospital, get chemotherapy, and go home and rest. The problem with that is you are constantly being reminded that you could die. On top of all that it's not like you get chemotherapy and have no side effects. You throw up, you lose your hair, you get mouth sores, you're in pain, you get the runs, you have sleepless nights, your bones feel like they are going to break, you have no energy, you are never hungry because everything you eat comes up, you're constantly having hot flashes, you get nauseous all the time and the list unfortunately goes on and on. It's hard to remain positive when all those things are happening to you every second of the day. You don't have the energy to do the things you used to do. It's hard to have conversations because of the chemo brain. You either lose all your weight or gain a lot of weight because of all the steroids you are taking. I started off in shape and semi-strong. Yes, I was itching myself 24/7 and I was losing weight but it was much easier dealing with that then the alternative. Now throughout my journey not every chemotherapy was like that fortunately but the majority were. You find yourself thinking, *Is it even worth it to go through the treatment?* You think maybe you should spend your last days traveling the world or doing whatever it is that you wanted before you die. The thing with myself is that for the first time in my life, at such a young age, I had to figure out how to survive and get through this so I could move on with my life. It was the toughest thing I've ever had to deal with and every day a new thing would happen and I would have to adapt.

Quite frankly, I knew it would be difficult but it was a million times harder than I could imagine. Those first few years I was suffering so much. I stopped going to school. My friends were in college and we all just lost touch. I didn't graduate college or anything like that.

After my cancer came back for the second time, I pushed myself to do something that I could pour my passion into. That's when I picked up boxing and I was so blessed to have the courage to do it. Yes, I was in pain all the time. Yes, my lungs were god-awful. Yes, I was anxious, nauseous, and all that all the time. But I pushed myself so hard to get out the front door and drive myself to the gym. I was so angry from all my suffering but instead of complaining and giving up I found something that made me feel better.

Finally, cancer helped me to be more ambitious than I used to be. Now mind you, I was always ambitious but now it's totally on another level. I know how precious life is and how we only get one shot. I've proved everyone wrong over the years and that's why I've become this way. Why should I tell myself I can't travel? I can't be an author? I can't be an athlete? I can't be a speaker? I can't have a business? I can be and do these things! I want it all and every day I do something productive to bring me closer to my goals. At the end of each day, I make a plan for the next day.

Almost dying was a major wake-up call that completely shifted my perspective on how I view life. When I was a boxer while I was battling cancer, my vitals were terrible. I had 50% lung functioning and I was so sick. When I lost in the ring, I didn't tell myself it was because I couldn't breathe. I didn't tell myself it was because I had chemotherapy this morning. I lost because I lost and there are no excuses. If you make no excuses, you work so much harder and it brings you so much closer to your goals. I'm so grateful for the lessons that cancer taught me. I was raised not to make excuses but, to be honest, it really kicked in when I got cancer. It teaches you how to get through things better, it teaches you how to be stronger because you're taking risks and trying to figure it all out. Through all my research on the topic of cancer for my communications class in college, I thought when I was diagnosed that I was just going to be in bed all day and I wouldn't amount to anything. But I was wrong. During my cancer journey I became an athlete, and I was able to tell my story to millions of people. Because of that, I was able to help and inspire so many.

My entire life I've always been ambitious because I know you only get one life. Even if I fail, at least I tried, and cancer has taught me that even if I fail, I need to get up and try again and keep doing it until I get it. Just like when my cancer got worse and worse. I kept trying different treatments until I found the one that works for the time frame. It's literally the same thing and when that treatment would work the relief I would get as well as my family was so big. Just like when I accomplish something I enjoy every second of it and it feels like a relief.

When I was growing up all my teachers thought I wouldn't amount to much in my life. That made me feel bad about myself and made me feel belittled. Later, my doctors told me I couldn't do this, I couldn't do that. They said I could never work out again, or box, or run. Well, the best thing you can do for me is tell me I can't do something. Every second of every day, no matter how tired or sick I am, I work my butt off to get the things I want. Throughout my cancer journey I've chosen not to allow anyone or anything make me feel belittled like I did when I was a kid. It is so hard beating cancer; I mean, it's by far the hardest thing I've ever had to do in my life. But I feel like I will beat this again. I've beaten cancer five times because I didn't make excuses, and cancer taught me that.

Chapter 25

HAPPY

"Quitting scares me the most because of how easy it is. So even though I am sick, I am happy to be in the fight."

What is it? What's the hardest thing I've ever had to learn or to fight to accomplish? Was it beating cancer five times? Was it that I was an athlete and lost my lifelong dream to compete in my sport? Was it getting through my anxiety disorders, like panic attacks, night terrors, and PTSD? Was it being in pain all the time? Was it watching my friends live their lives while mine became a battle in which success meant not dying each day? No way, that is the easy stuff.

For me, it was digging deeper than I ever thought possible. To the core of my soul to have that conversation with the part of myself that wants to be bitter and angry and to say "I quit." Instead, I have learned to push back with every ounce of will and to say, "No way will I quit!" The real battle has been finding a way to be happy in this difficult and seemingly unfair fight against a relentless foe, cancer. The pain, even when treated with medication, is severe and when it is not, its return is imminent and the anticipation is brutal. Sleeping, the time to escape and rest, the time in which the body typically recovers, is interrupted with so many thoughts and fears rushing through my mind. For me, an idle mind, even in a restful state, can truly be the devil's workshop.

Since I was first diagnosed at 19 years old, all I've ever wanted was a chance. Just like everyone else, I have dreams and goals. While the goalposts have moved due to my diagnosis, the outcome remains the same. I know I am here for a purpose and I want to be here to make a real difference in the lives of others.

Over the years, finding a way to be happy when there's always something wrong with my health is the epitome of pursuing an evasive goal. Beyond the chemo treatment, the radiation, the biopsies, the sickness, the fatigue, and the waiting for results of tests, scans, or blood work, the most difficult part but the most rewarding and fulfilling lesson I had to learn is to find a way to be happy. I've committed to appreciate and to focus on what I have. What? Yes, the real point is I am grateful that I can keep fighting. Every new day to fight is another day that I am alive. This has helped me be confident in the person I am. Even though I'm still in this state where every hour of every day I battle both mentally and physically, there are times of quiet and calm when I try to clear my head and reflect on the meaning and the why. It is in this precious place I started asking myself (and now tell myself) to find a way today to be happy. I am and it's the fight that gives me life!

The fight is more than just about surviving. I will have to fight for the rest of my life and the battle has taught me that fighting actually gives me life and a deeper meaning. I don't know what my future holds, so every day I seek nuggets of "in the moment" opportunity. Little wins not just for me, but maybe for that family that has just been impacted by a cancer diagnosis. They call me looking for understanding, hope, and strength. My staying in the fight gives me the energy to be an example, and maybe that bit of light in a dark place is worth everything.

So you might be reading this and wondering, "Where did this motivation come from? Is it real or just some mental babble?" Trust me, it is very real. It all started one morning when I woke up and went outside.

I was feeling pretty good that morning. It was a moment of no stress, no pain, no itching, no anxiety. I looked at the rising sun, took a deep breath, and closed my eyes. When I opened them, I felt free! Free from wanting, wishing, anger, disappointment. Free from the fear of what's next or the uncertainty of the unknown. This made the fight not about the outcome, but about my unwillingness to quit. Being here with the ability to fight beats not being here at all. Next round? Bring it!

I fight because if I don't fight, nothing gets better. If I don't fight there is no chance of reaching any goal. Yes, it's hard, whether going through cancer or depression or maybe the loss of a loved one or enduring a professional challenge or the struggle of a difficult relationship. I look at my pain as a reminder that I have the opportunity to be stronger TODAY. How can I deal with today, be the best version of myself, and be an example for anyone fighting their own battle? When I realized that staying in the battle has an impact beyond me, I realized the ripple is real. If we can have an influence and be a spark of encouragement by what others see in our journey, the energy returns in waves.

When you make the conscious choice to have a better life and you fight for it, I believe in my heart that whatever you are going through, you will get through it. There was a point when I was confined to a wheelchair when I couldn't do a single push-up, nor even go to the bathroom on my own. I was at a point where death was an option that could have ended the pain of the fight. Somehow, I said no. So it's just understanding that if you hold on, if you can take steps of even an inch at a time, it will get better.

You just have to be the one to make the decision. You commit to fighting today. Some days you might not be able to. But you must remind yourself every day when you wake up to keep going. The first thing I say when I start my day is, "BRING IT!" I tell myself that anything can happen at any point today. The beauty is that I have a choice. I have learned to choose HAPPY! You can too. Thank you. I have to go; I am late for treatment. No worries, it's just chemo.

QUOTES I LIVE BY

"And so rock bottom became the solid foundation on which I rebuilt my life." – J.K. Rowling

"I want the world to be a better place because I was here" - Will Smith

"Strength and growth come only through continuous effort and struggle." - Napoleon Hill

"The key to immortality is first living a life worth remembering." - Bruce Lee

"We cannot change the cards we are dealt, just how we play the hand." - Randy Pausch

"I am more than my scars." - Andrew Davidson

"If you can look up, you can get up." - Eric Thomas

"Grow through what you go through."

"I don't take steps back in my life, I always move forward. If I can't move forward, I pivot."

"You know, Donkey, things are more than what they seem." – Shrek

ACKNOWLEDGEMENTS

Being an author has been a dream of mine for quite some time, so it makes the most sense to thank the people that made this possible. The first person I want to thank is **Helen Demestihas**. Helen and I have been through a lot together. She's helped me spread my story in so many ways and I'll be forever grateful for it all. Helen is like family to me. She's always someone I could go to for anything, including finding the best writer in such a short period of time. **Tammy Kling**, an amazing writer, has a gift of telling someone's story. Her professionalism and talent come second to how compassionate and empathetic she is. I'll be forever grateful for the gift she has given me.

There are so many people that have helped me on my journey since I was 19 years old. **Allison Moskowitz**, my oncologist, has always been there and has never given up on me. Whether it was the late-night calls or finding out results of my scans and so much more, she's been there through it all. I've had a lot of therapists over the years, but since I was diagnosed with PTSD, **Michael Rosenthal** has always gone the extra mile for me. He's someone I feel comfortable telling everything to and he has become a friend to me. Because of everything I've been through, I've suffered physically in many ways. **Robin J. Iversen,** has helped me through my everyday pain. With the pain I go through, sometimes it feels like it will never get any better, and she is the person who makes me feel like things will get better. **Dr. Mohamed Tantawi** and **Dr. Mona Tantawi** have handled my pediatric care with grace for so many years.

I was an athlete my entire life and when I got sick, I made the decision that not only did I want to remain an athlete but I wanted to push myself to do something that I never thought possible. The two sports I chose to do were boxing and being a strongman athlete. Both coaches, **Burt and Frank,** always pushed me and never treated me any differently from anybody else. It was that training that, every time I went to bed, I didn't feel like I was going to die.

Kelly Conheeney, thank you for always pushing me and believing in me.

Brendan Walsh, out of all the friends that I've had in my entire life, you were by far the greatest one I've ever had. No matter what was going on, you were always there through the good, the bad, the ugly. At times, I may not have been the greatest friend, but I always tried my best. Thank you for it all.

Bruce Pulver, the first time we ever talked was to prepare for the interview you were going to give me. I immediately knew from our first call that I was going to be friends with you for the rest of my life. When I chose to add more to my book, you made my words flow with ease and helped my message get across in ways I couldn't do on my own. I hope one day to be on stage with you and to be able to speak together. You're one of the greatest people I have ever met in my life. BOOK: *Above The Chatter, Our Words Matter*

www.abovethechatterourwordsmatter.com

To **my aunts and uncles**, thank you for always believing in me, through my cancer, through my life, and knowing I could be anything.

Katharina Harf, we met years ago when I needed a match. You gave me my first opportunity to tell my story to an audience. It was after that speech that I knew what I wanted to do for the rest of my life. What was even better than all the things we did together is that I look at you as family. From the first moment I met you, I knew we were going to be in each other's lives for the rest of time. There will always be a special place in my heart for you.

Bradley Cooper, right off the bat, I knew we would always be close friends. It's difficult being sick for so long and you lose opportunities to do special things. If I had to look at the coolest things I've ever done in my life, most of them are with you. Even though you're always so busy, you always have found time to talk to me and my family. Thank you for the memories.

Laura Furlipa, thank you for it all. No matter what is was. When it happened. You were always there and I'll be forever grateful.

Ann Tatlock, I got in contact with you toward the end of this process. What a pleasure it was to work with you and also become friends at the same time!

Nanny and Grandpa, you always believed in me. You always loved me. My best memories of being a kid are with you. You're the best grandparents anyone could ever ask for. I love you with all my heart.

My brothers, **Vincent and Michael**. Growing up, my job was to look after both of you. Once I got sick, the roles changed, and you both looked after me. I've been so proud of both of you, and you've turned out to be the best brothers anyone could ask for. Michael, I know there's a part of you that doesn't think this, but what you did by donating for my stem cell transplant is why I'm alive today. I promise that I'm not going anywhere, and I will be everything that I've said I was going to be. Whether you know this or not, I am prouder to be your older brother then you could possibly imagine. You've become so strong, and I believe in my heart you will be everything you always dreamed of. You've always inspired me to be better. Every time I wanted to quit, I always thought of our family, and it made me continue to hold on and keep going. Vincent, I don't even know where to begin to thank you. There's is no me without you. I would never have gotten this far without you. You sacrificed close to half of your life to make sure I have a life. You always have put me first. Whether it's driving me to appointments or being there for everything I've done, I can't think of a single memory of something I'm proud of where you aren't there. There are just no words to say thank you for what you did for me and our family, while at the same time accomplishing the things you've done. I believe in you because of how strong you are. Both you and Michael are the reasons I didn't quit. You are the reasons I push myself in every aspect of my life. You inspire me and at the same time I'm as strong as I am because of you. No matter what happens, I will always be your big brother and I will always be in your heart. I love you.

Mom and Dad, you are what every parent should strive to be. The lessons I've learned from you are why I am the man I am today. Dad, as a kid the only person I wanted to be was you. Through all the pain and all the suffering, you were there for me. You were there for every hockey game, every doctor appointment, I mean everything. When I knew I needed to be strong and I didn't know how, I looked at you and Mom and saw what you did. You always pushed me to be stronger, to be better, and you taught me that there are no excuses in this world, and nobody owes you anything. You found a way to be tough on me, but always knew how to make me feel better. There's so much I want to thank you for and there aren't enough words to say how thankful I am. Thank you for teaching me how to be a man. Thank you for being by my side, and more importantly thank you for being my dad. The last person I want to thank is the person that means more to me than anyone in this world, my mom. You and dad always did everything for us. And you would be whatever it is that we needed. I needed a superhero to get through this and, Mom, you knew I needed one, so you became one. I'm sorry for the pain I've caused you through my battle. But you are my best friend. I'm alive because of you and Dad, and of course my brothers. All the calls, doctor visits, the list goes on and on. You never gave up on me my entire life. You always pushed me, you always loved me. You're my best friend and without you I wouldn't be here. Thank you for all the memories, I love you and Dad with all my heart, and I will keep fighting no matter what happens. I love you.